PocketRadiologist™
Musculoskeletal
100 Top Diagnoses

PocketRadiologist™
Musculoskeletal
100 Top Diagnoses

David W Stoller MD
Director, California Advanced Imaging and MRI
California Pacific Medical Center
San Francisco, California

Director, National Orthopaedic Imaging Associates
San Francisco, California

Phillip F J Tirman MD
National Orthopedic Imaging Associates
Greenbrae, California

Co-director, Musculoskeletal MRI
California Pacific Medical Center
San Francisco, California

Miriam A Bredella MD
Department of Radiology
University of California San Francisco
San Francisco, California

Research contribution: *Gen Maruyama MD*
                           Jana Crain MD

With 200 drawings and radiographic images

Drawings: *Salvador Beltran MD*
                   Lane R Bennion MS
                   James A Cooper MD
Image Editing: *Ming Q Huang MD*
                   Melissa Petersen

AMIRSYS

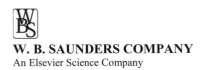

W. B. SAUNDERS COMPANY
An Elsevier Science Company

AMIRSYS

A medical reference publishing company

First Edition

Text – Copyright David W Stoller MD 2002

Drawings - Copyright Amirsys Inc 2002

Compilation - Copyright Amirsys Inc 2002

Composition by Amirsys Inc, Salt Lake City, Utah

Printed by K/P Corp, Salt Lake City, Utah

ISBN: 0-7216-9701-1

Preface

The **PocketRadiologist**™ series is an innovative, quick reference designed to deliver succinct, up-to-date information to practicing professionals "at the point of service." As close as your pocket, each title in the series is written by world-renowned authors, specialists in their area. These experts have designated the "top 100" diagnoses in every major body area, bulleted the most essential facts, and offered high-resolution imaging to illustrate each topic. Selected references are included for further review. Full color anatomic-pathologic computer graphics model many of the actual diseases.

Each **PocketRadiologist**™ title follows an identical format. The same information is in the same place—every time—and takes you quickly from key facts to imaging findings, differential diagnosis, pathology, pathophysiology, and relevant clinical information.

PocketRadiologist™ titles are available in both print and hand-held PDA formats. Our first modules feature Brain, Head and Neck, and Orthopedic (Musculoskeletal) Imaging. Additional titles include Spine and Cord, Chest, Breast, Vascular, Cardiac, Pediatrics, Emergency, and Genital Urinary, and Gastro Intestinal. Enjoy!

Anne G Osborn MD
Editor-in-Chief, Amirsys Inc

PocketRadiologist™
Musculoskeletal
Top 100 Diagnoses

The diagnoses in this book are divided into 9 sections in the following order:

Shoulder
Elbow
Wrist and Hand
Hip
Knee
Ankle and Foot
Bone Marrow
Bone Tumors
Soft Tissue Tumors

Table of Diagnoses

Soft Tissue Tumors

Notice and Disclaimer

The information in this product ("Product") is provided as a reference for use by licensed medical professionals and no others. It does not and should not be construed as any form of medical diagnosis or professional medical advice on any matter. Receipt or use of this Product, in whole or in part, does not constitute or create a doctor-patient, therapist-patient, or other healthcare professional relationship between Amirsys Inc. ("Amirsys") and any recipient. This Product may not reflect the most current medical developments, and Amirsys makes no claims, promises, or guarantees about accuracy, completeness, or adequacy of the information contained in or linked to the Product. The Product is not a substitute for or replacement of professional medical judgment. Amirsys and its affiliates, authors, contributors, partners, and sponsors disclaim all liability or responsibility for any injury and/or damage to persons or property in respect to actions taken or not taken based on any and all Product information.

In the cases where drugs or other chemicals are prescribed, readers are advised to check the Product information currently provided by the manufacturer of each drug to be administered to verify the recommended dose, the method and duration of administration, and contraindications. It is the responsibility of the treating physician relying on experience and knowledge of the patient to determine dosages and the best treatment for the patient.

To the maximum extent permitted by applicable law, Amirsys provides the Product AS IS AND WITH ALL FAULTS, AND HEREBY DISCLAIMS ALL WARRANTIES AND CONDITIONS, WHETHER EXPRESS, IMPLIED OR STATUTORY, INCLUDING BUT NOT LIMITED TO, ANY (IF ANY) IMPLIED WARRANTIES OR CONDITIONS OF MERCHANTABILITY, OF FITNESS FOR A PARTICULAR PURPOSE, OF LACK OF VIRUSES, OR ACCURACY OR COMPLETENESS OF RESPONSES, OR RESULTS, AND OF LACK OF NEGLIGENCE OR LACK OF WORKMANLIKE EFFORT. ALSO, THERE IS NO WARRANTY OR CONDITION OF TITLE, QUIET ENJOYMENT, QUIET POSSESSION, CORRESPONDENCE TO DESCRIPTION OR NON-INFRINGEMENT, WITH REGARD TO THE PRODUCT. THE ENTIRE RISK AS TO THE QUALITY OF OR ARISING OUT OF USE OR PERFORMANCE OF THE PRODUCT REMAINS WITH THE READER.

Amirsys disclaims all warranties of any kind if the Product was customized, repackaged or altered in any way by any third party.

PocketRadiologist™
Musculoskeletal
100 Top Diagnoses

SHOULDER

Rotator Cuff Tendinopathy

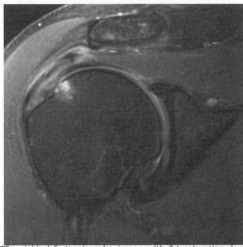

A coronal T2-weighted fast spin echo image with fat saturation demonstrates a heterogeneous mildly thickened supraspinatus tendon consistent with tendinosis with mild reactive subacromial bursitis present.

Key Facts
- Overuse degeneration and tearing of the rotator cuff
- May occur secondary to impingement or acute trauma
- Most common reason for MRI referral of the shoulder
- May be painful even without tendon tear

Imaging Findings
MR Findings
- Increased signal intensity on all pulse sequences
- Tendon usually thickened
- Tendon often inhomogeneous
- Partial tear seen as fluid entering tendon but only part of the way through
- Through-and-through (full thickness) tear demonstrated as fluid extending through gap in tendon with variable retraction
- Full thickness tear may be associated with fatty atrophy of the muscles in chronic cases
- Tears best seen on coronal and sagittal images

Differential Diagnosis
Calcific Tendinitis
- Tendon may be thickened and is often decreased in signal intensity
Intratendinous Cyst
- Thickened tendon but cyst is visible on T2-weighted images
- Associated with partial tear of rotator cuff

Pathology
General
- Etiology-Pathogenesis
  - Overuse degeneration and tearing of the rotator cuff

Rotator Cuff Tendinopathy

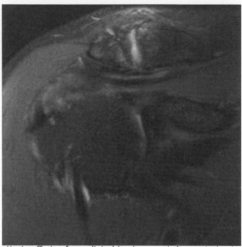

A 2nd patient suffering from clinical impingement demonstrates tendinosis.

○ Most commonly secondary to impingement syndrome (curved acromion plus overuse)
○ Can occur in collagen vascular diseases along with tendinosis of other tendons
○ May occur acutely but usually in the setting of preexisting tendinosis

Gross Pathologic or Surgical Features
• Usually thickened, indurated tendon
• Break in integrity of tendon in partially torn and torn tendons
• Partial tear may be bursal surface, articular surface or interstitial

Microscopic Features
• Collagen degeneration without significant influx of inflammatory cells: "Tendinosis" is preferred term over tendinitis
• Break in integrity of tendon in partially torn (bursal, articular or interstitial) and through-and-through torn tendons
• Fatty infiltration of muscle tissue in chronically torn tendons

Clinical Issues
Presentation
• Insidious onset of pain in adult patient with impingement syndrome
• Pain in the setting of athletics in the case of internal impingement: Younger patient
• Peak age 40 and above for impingement
• Posttraumatic continued pain

Treatment & Prognosis
• Physical therapy
• Subacromial decompression for impingement

Selected References
1. Gartsman GM: Arthroscopic management of rotator cuff disease. J Am Acad Orthop Surg. 6(4): 259-66, 1998
2. Fritz RC et al: MR imaging of the rotator cuff. Magn Reson Imaging Clin N Am. 5(4): 735-54, 1997
3. Neer CD et al: Cuff-tear arthropathy. J Bone Joint Surg. 65(9): 1232-44, 1983

Rotator Cuff Full Thickness Tear

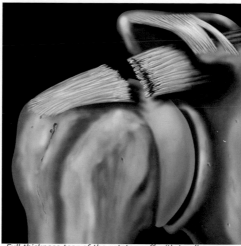

Full thickness tear of the rotator cuff with tendinous gap.

Key Facts
- Overuse degeneration and complete tearing of the rotator cuff
- May occur secondary to impingement or acute trauma
- Seen as interruption of the decreased signal intensity tendon usually involving the distal tendon anteriorly or sometimes involving the relatively avascular "critical zone"

Imaging Findings
General Features
- A tear or gap in the tendon which can become filled with joint or bursal fluid or granulation tissue

MR Findings
- Fluid signal intensity filling a gap in the tendon which is best seen with fat saturated fast spin echo T2-weighted images
- Variable retraction and degeneration of the tendon edges seen
- Full thickness tear may be associated with fatty atrophy of the muscles in chronic cases
- Tears best seen on coronal and sagittal images
- Associated with fluid (increased signal intensity on fat saturated fast spin echo T2-weighted images) with the subacromial bursa
- Associated with fluid within the subcoracoid bursa especially with anterior supraspinatus tears and rotator interval tears

Other Modality Findings
- Plain film arthrograms and MR arthrograms demonstrate fluid extravasating from the joint into the subacromial bursa after contrast injection

Differential Diagnosis
Intratendinous Cyst
- Thickened tendon but cyst is visible on T2-weighted images

Rotator Cuff Full Thickness Tear

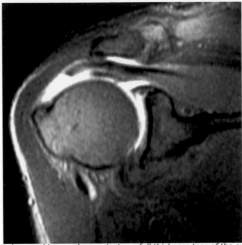

A T2-weighted coronal image demonstrates a full thickness tear of the supraspinatus tendon with retraction.

<u>Partial Tear of Rotator Cuff</u>
- Fluid within but not through-and-through the tendon

Pathology
<u>General</u>
- Etiology-Pathogenesis
  - Overuse degeneration and complete tearing of the rotator cuff
  - Most commonly secondary to Impingement Syndrome (curved acromion plus overuse)
  - Can occur in collagen vascular diseases along with tears of other tendons
  - May occur acutely but usually in the setting of preexisting tendinosis

<u>Gross Pathologic or Surgical Features</u>
- Usually thickened, indurated tendon edges
- Break in integrity of tendon

<u>Microscopic Features</u>
- Break in integrity of tendon
- Preexisting collagen degeneration without significant influx of inflammatory cells: "Tendinosis" is preferred term over tendinitis
- Fatty infiltration of muscle tissue in chronically torn tendons

Clinical Issues
<u>Presentation</u>
- Peak age 40 and above especially for impingement
- Insidious onset of pain in adult patient with impingement syndrome
- Pain in the setting of athletics in the case of internal impingement – younger patient
- Posttraumatic continued pain

Rotator Cuff Full Thickness Tear

Treatment & Prognosis
- Depends on level of activity and cause of tear
- Impingement: Usually subacromial decompression (acromioplasty) and tendon repair unless massive cuff tear or those associated with atrophy
- Massive cuff tears and those associated with atrophy treated with debridement

Selected References
1. Handelberg FW: Treatment options in full thickness rotator cuff tears. Acta Orthop Belg. 67(2): 110-5, 2001
2. Murrell GA et al: Diagnosis of rotator cuff tears. Lancet. 357(9258): 769-70, 2001
3. Stoller DW et al: The Shoulder, in Magnetic Resonance Imaging in Orthopaedics and Sports Medicine. J.B. Lippincott: Philadelphia. 597-742, 1997

Subscapularis Rupture

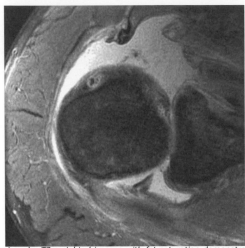

Axial fast spin echo T2-weighted images with fat saturation demonstrate complete rupture of the subscapularis tendon with retraction in a patient who suffered from an acute anterior dislocation.

Key Facts
- Occurs secondary to anterior dislocation in patients generally older than 40 years of age
- Occurs secondary to posterior dislocation in any age

Imaging Findings
MR Findings
- Increased signal intensity on all pulse sequences
- Tendon often inhomogeneous
- Partial tear seen as fluid entering tendon but only part of the way through
- Through-and-through (full thickness) tear demonstrated as fluid extending through gap in tendon with variable retraction: Best seen on axial images

Plain Film Findings
- Lesser tuberosity fracture on plain films

Differential Diagnosis
Tendinosis without Rupture
- In this case a gap is not visualized and the history is usually not present

Pathology
General
- Etiology-Pathogenesis
  - May be sole tendon torn after anterior dislocation especially in older patients
  - May occur with or without an avulsion of the lesser tuberosity in a patient after posterior dislocation

Gross Pathology or Surgical Features
- Break in integrity of tendon in partially torn and torn tendons

Subscapularis Rupture

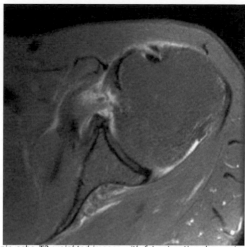

Axial fast spin echo T2 weighted images with fat saturation demonstrate complete rupture of the subscapularis tendon with retraction in a patient who suffered from an acute anterior dislocation.

Microscopic Features
- Break in integrity of tendon in partially torn and through-and-through torn tendons
- Fatty infiltration of muscle tissue in chronically torn tendons

Clinical Issues

Presentation
- Patient over approximately forty years of age presenting with first time anterior dislocation
- Occurs secondary to posterior dislocation in any age
- Clinical positive lift-off test (inability to lift hand against resistance from the small of the back)
- May occur secondary to posterior dislocation especially in the case of tonic-clonic seizures
- May be misdiagnosed clinically as an axillary neuropraxis

Treatment & Prognosis
- Open surgical repair

Selected References
1. Tirman et al: Humeral avulsion of the anterior shoulder stabilizing structures after anterior shoulder dislocation: Demonstration by MRI and MR arthrography. Skeletal Radiol. 25(8): 743-8, 1996
2. Neviaser RJ et al: Recurrent instability of the shoulder after age 40. J Shoulder Elbow Surg. 4(6): 416-8, 1995
3. Patten RM: Tears of the anterior portion of the rotator cuff (the subscapularis tendon): MR imaging findings. AJR Am J Roentgenol. 162(2): 351-4, 1994

Acromioclavicular Arthrosis

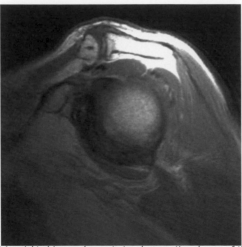

A sagittal T 1-weighted image demonstrates degenerative change of the A-C joint with inferiorly directed osteophytes.

Key Facts
- Common cause of anterosuperior shoulder pain
- Often accompanies rotator cuff disease in the elderly

Imaging Findings
General Features
- Chondromalacia
- Distal clavicular and/or proximal acromial cysts and edema
- Synovitis
- Subchondral sclerosis
- Periarticular edema

Differential Diagnosis
Post Traumatic Osteolysis
- History of trauma often weight lifting
- Variable degrees of edema and clavicular destruction
Degenerative Changes of an Os Acromiale
- Occurs between the os acromiale and the remaining acromion
- Usually slightly lateral and posterior to A-C joint
Impingement
- Pain anteriorly with abduction
- Lidocaine injection into A-C joint may help differentiate

Pathology
General
- Etiology-Pathogenesis
  - Adult or athlete
  - May occur secondary to acromioclavicular separation or as typical degenerative change

Acromioclavicular Arthrosis

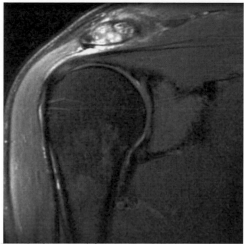

A coronal T2-weighted image with fat saturation demonstrates degenerative changes consisting of edema, synovitis and subarticular cyst formation.

Gross Pathologic or Surgical Features
• Osteoarthritic changes consisting of chondromalacia, synovitis, subchondral sclerosis, periarticular edema, and distal clavicular and/or proximal acromial cysts and edema

Microscopic Features
• Degenerative arthritis with variable amounts of inflammatory cells, chondral degeneration, subarticular geodes, and subchondral osteocytic build-up (sclerosis)

Clinical Issues

Presentation
• Adult
• Anterior superior pain
• Positive cross-body or horizontal adduction test
• Positive lidocaine injection test

Treatment & Prognosis
• Non-steroidal anti-inflammatory drugs, physical therapy
• Mumford procedure for advanced cases

Selected References
1. Stein BE et al: Detection of acromioclavicular joint pathology in asymptomatic shoulders with magnetic resonance imaging. J Shoulder Elbow Surg. 10(3): 204-8, 2001
2. Clarke HD et al: Acromioclavicular joint injuries. Orthop Clin North Am. 31(2): 177-87, 2000
3. Shaffer BS: Painful conditions of the acromioclavicular joint. J Am Acad Orthop Surg. 7(3): 176-88, 1999

Subacromial Impingement

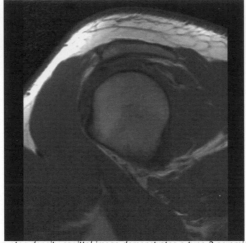

A proton density sagittal image demonstrates a type 3 acromion.

Key Facts
- Progressively painful compression of the supraspinatus tendon and subacromial bursa between the humeral head and the coracoacromial arch
- Caused by repeated microtrauma of curved acromion on rotator cuff
- Most common reason for obtaining MRI of the shoulder

Imaging Findings
MR Findings
- Type II (curved) or type III (anterior inferiorly hooked) acromion process predisposes
- Enthesophyte formation underneath acromion predisposes
- Lateral downsloping predisposes
- Thickened heterogeneous tendon or torn tendon
- Fluid in subacromial bursa is common

Differential Diagnosis
Torn Cuff or Tendinopathy
- In the absence of a curved acromion
Internal Impingement
Acute Trauma
Os Acromiale
- Degenerative changes may lead to pain with abduction
Suprascapular Denervation
- May mimic impingement clinically because of weakness and pain of supraspinatus and infraspinatus
Adhesive Capsulitis
- Limitation in both active and passive range of motion whereas impingement patients usually don't have limitation in passive range of motion
- Usually visualize thickened edematous capsule on fat saturated axial Proton density or T2-weighted images

Subacromial Impingement

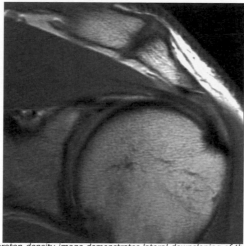

A coronal proton density image demonstrates lateral downsloping of the acromion.

Aging and Degeneration
- Impingement may play a role

Arthritides and Systemic Disorders
- Rheumatoid arthritis, diabetes, and renal disease weaken tendons elsewhere

Pathology

General
- Etiology-Pathogenesis
  o Caused by repeated microtrauma of curved acromion on rotator cuff
  o Associated with type II and type III acromion
  o Common in active adults or occupations including overhead-type activities

Gross Pathologic or Surgical Features
- Type II (curved) or type III (anterior inferiorly hooked) acromion process commonly found
- Enthesophyte formation underneath acromion commonly found
- Lateral downsloping commonly found

Microscopic Features
- Collagen degeneration in the setting of intermittent inflammatory tendinitis
- Hypertrophic and inflammatory bursitis common

Staging or Grading Criteria
- Stage I: Reversible edema and hemorrhage typically in active patient 25 years of age or younger
- Stage II: Fibrosis and tendinitis
- Stage III: Degeneration and rupture often associated with osseous changes most commonly in patients over 40 years of age

Subacromial Impingement

Clinical Issues
<u>Presentation</u>
- Adult
- Young athletes participating in sports requiring overhead arm movements
- Insidious onset of pain
- Pain to palpation of the rotator cuff within the range of extension
- Range of motion often preserved
- May have painful arc of motion
- Pain and weakness to supraspinatus testing is often present

<u>Treatment & Prognosis</u>
- Initial treatment is conservative predominantly of physical therapy
- Steriod injections are commonly given
- Recalcitrant cases are treated with sunacromial decompression/ acromioplasty

Selected References
1. Fritz RC et al: MR imaging of the rotator cuff. Magn Reson Imaging Clin N Am. 5(4): 735-54, 1997
2. Neer CS: Impingement lesions. Clin. Orthop. 1983. 173:70-7, 1983
3. Neer CS: Anterior acromioplasty for the chronic impingement syndrome in the shoulder. J Bone Joint Surg. 54A: 41-50, 1972

SLAP Lesions

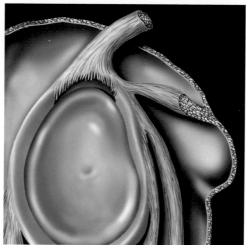

SLAP II lesion with avulsion of the superior labrum and biceps anchor.

Key Facts
- Tear of the superior labrum extending from anterior to the biceps anchor to posterior to it

Imaging Findings
MR Findings
- Fluid signal intensity within the superior labrum at the biceps anchor on T2-weighted images
- Detached fragment of labrum
- Globular high signal on short TE images
- Irregularity and/or widening of recess beneath the superior labrum

Differential Diagnosis
Impingement
- Some clinical signs may mimic impingement since the long head of the biceps is involved in both
Sublabral Hole
- At imaging the anterior superior labrum is detached often in both
- Sublabral hole confined to anterior superior labrum and SLAP involves biceps anchor
Buford Complex
- Buford complex confined to anterior superior labrum and SLAP involves biceps anchor

Pathology
General
- Etiology-Pathogenesis
  - Tear of the glenoid labrum involving the biceps anchor
  - Most often posttraumatic
  - May occur secondary to overhead racquet sports

SLAP Lesions

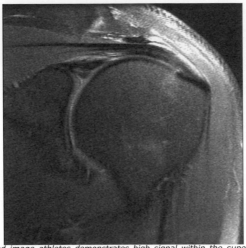

T2-weighted image athletes demonstrates high signal within the superior labrum consistent with a SLAP lesion.

Gross Pathologic or Surgical Features
- Degenerative fraying or frank tears of the superior labrum/biceps anchor

Microscopic Features
- Fibrocartilaginous degeneration and/or tear of the superior labrum/ biceps anchor

Staging or Grading Criteria
- Type I: Degenerative fraying
- Type II: Detachment of the biceps anchor and superior labrum
- Type III: Bucket handle tear of the superior labrum leaving the biceps still attached to the underlying glenoid
- Type IV: Bucket handle tear extending into the biceps
- Type V: Bankart lesion which dissects upward to involve the biceps anchor
- Type VI: Unstable radial or flap tears which involve separation of the biceps anchor
- Type VII: Extension of a superior labral tear to involve the middle glenohumeral ligament
- Type VIII: Equals type II SLAP + entire posterior labral tear: Anterior inferior labrum is normal.
- Type IX: Circumferential labral tear

Clinical Issues

Presentation
- Posttraumatic patient with only approximately one-third with symptoms referable to the biceps tendon
- Patient status post traction injury (forced extension on flexed forearm), typically type II
- Patient status post fall on outstretched hand (31%), usually type III, IV or V lesion
- Patient status post anterior dislocation (16%), often a type V

SLAP Lesions

<u>Treatment & Prognosis</u>
- Debridement and / or arthroscopic repair

Selected References
1. Musgrave DS et al: SLAP lesions: current concepts. Am J Orthop 30(1): 29-38, 2001
2. Bencardino JT et al: Superior labrum anterior-posterior lesions: diagnosis with MR arthrography of the shoulder. Radiology. 214(1): 267-71, 2001
3. Snyder SJ et al: SLAP lesions of the shoulder. Arthroscopy. 6(4): 274-9, 1990

Bankart Lesion

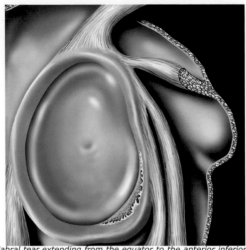

Anterior labral tear extending from the equator to the anterior inferior quadrant.

Key Facts
- Avulsion of the inferior glenohumeral labral ligamentous attachment to the glenoid after anterior dislocation of the shoulder
- The scapular periosteum is disrupted
- Cause of recurrent instability if improper healing of initial lesion occurs

Imaging Findings
MR Findings
- Detachment of the inferior glenohumeral ligament and labrum from the underlying glenoid
- Labrum may be discretely torn or markedly heterogeneous and predominantly of increased signal intensity on axial images
- In chronic case the lesion may be partially healed and fibrosed giving the appearance of heterogeneous but predominantly decreased signal intensity on all pulse sequences
- Often accompanied by edema and hemorrhage (increased signal on T2 weighted images) in surrounding soft tissues
- May be accompanied by a fracture of the underlying glenoid: Increased signal intensity on T2 weighted images and visible fracture line with variable degrees of distraction
- Detached labrum at ABER imaging
- Torn, distracted labrum on coronal images

Differential Diagnosis
Bankart Variation Lesion
- Perthes, ALSPA lesions
Intact Periosteum
- Often difficult to accurately diagnose at MRI
Partially Torn Non-Distracted Labrum after Subluxation

Bankart Lesion

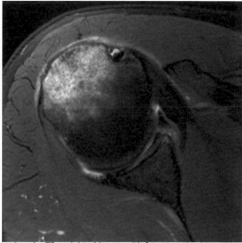

An axial fast spin echo T2-weighted image with fat saturation in a patient status post acute anterior dislocation demonstrates a torn labrum, disruption of the labral attachment to the glenoid, a bone trabecular injury of the anterior glenoid rim and an acute trabecular injury of the humerus.

Pathology
General
- Etiology-Pathogenesis
  - Most common lesion to occur after initial anterior dislocation of the shoulder in a patient under 40 years of age

Gross Pathologic or Surgical Features
- Avulsion of the inferior glenohumeral labral ligamentous attachment to the glenoid after anterior dislocation of the shoulder
- Accompanied by osteochondral fracture in some cases

Microscopic Features
- Hemorrhagic, torn, fibrocartilaginous labrum with variable degrees of fibrosis depending on chronicity

Clinical Issues
Presentation
- Typically younger patient (under 40 years) status post anterior dislocation (single or multiple dislocations)
- Positive apprehension test in patients with recurrent instability

Treatment & Prognosis
- Conservative with a sling to allow healing
- Surgical or arthroscopic repair for repeat dislocations

Selected References
1. Gartsman GM et al: Arthroscopic treatment of anterior-inferior glenohumeral instability. Two to five-year follow-up. J Bone Joint Surg Am 82 A (7): 991-1003, 2000
2. Burkhart SS et al: Traumatic glenohumeral bone defects and their relationship to failure of arthroscopic Bankart repairs: Significance of the inverted-pear glenoid and the humeral engaging Hill-Sachs lesion. Arthroscopy. 16(7): 677-94, 2000
3. Tirman PF et al: A practical approach to imaging of the shoulder with emphasis on MR imaging, Orthop Clin North Am. 28(4): 483-515, 1997

Bankart Variation Lesions

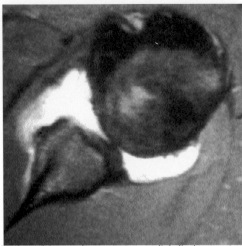

A T2-weighted axial image demonstrates medial displacement of the labral ligamentous complex along the scapular neck. The patient was immediately status post dislocation that resulted in the large effusion.

Key Facts
- Avulsion of the inferior glenohumeral labral ligamentous attachment to the glenoid after anterior dislocation of the shoulder
- The scapular periosteum is intact
- The labral ligamentous complex is displaced medially in the ALPSA lesion (Anterior Labroligamentous Periosteal Sleeve Avulsion Lesion)
- The labral ligamentous complex is nondisplaced in neutral positioning but non-attached in the Perthes lesion
- Cause of recurrent instability if improper healing of initial lesion occurs

Imaging Findings
MR Findings
- Detachment and medial displacement of the inferior glenohumeral ligament and labrum from the underlying glenoid (ALPSA)
- Usually normal positioning of the inferior glenohumeral ligament and labrum from the underlying glenoid (Perthes)
- Labrum may be normal in appearance or heterogeneous and predominantly of increased signal intensity on axial images
- In chronic case the lesion may be partially healed and fibrosed giving the appearance of heterogeneous but predominantly decreased signal intensity on all pulse sequences
- Often accompanied by edema and hemorrhage (increased signal on T2-weighted images) in surrounding soft tissues in acute cases
- May be accompanied by a fracture of the underlying glenoid: Increased signal intensity on T2-weighted images and visible fracture line with variable degrees of distraction
- Detached labrum at ABER imaging with the Perthes lesion
- Medially displaced labrum on coronal images

Bankart Variation Lesions

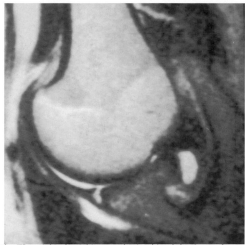

Fast spin echo T2-weighted axial image obtained in abduction and external rotation demonstrates detachment of the labral ligamentous complex from the anterior glenoid. The scapular periosteum is intact.

Differential Diagnosis
Bankart Lesion
- Disrupted periosteum with the Bankart lesion which is often difficult to accurately diagnose at MRI

Partially Torn Non-Detached Labrum after Subluxation

Pathology
General
- Etiology-Pathogenesis
  - Generally occurs after initial anterior dislocation of the shoulder in a patient under 40 years of age

Gross Pathologic or Surgical Features
- Avulsion of the inferior glenohumeral labral ligamentous attachment to the glenoid after anterior dislocation of the shoulder
- Medial displacement (ALPSA) with fibrosis and resynovialization in chronic cases
- Both lesions can appear remarkably normal at arthroscopy especially in the chronic state
- Accompanied by osteochondral fracture in some cases

Microscopic Features
- Hemorrhagic, torn, fibrocartilaginous labrum with variable degrees of fibrosis depending on chronicity

Clinical Presentation
- Typically younger patient (under 40 years) status post anterior dislocation (single or multiple dislocations)

Treatment & Prognosis
- ALPSA lesions are mobilized surgically or arthroscopically so that the normal anatomy is reapproximated and then repaired

Selected References

1. Cvitanic OP et al: Using abduction and external rotation of the shoulder to increase the sensitivity of MR arthrography in revealing tears of the anterior glenoid labrum. AJR Am J Roentgenol. 169(3): 837-44, 1997
2. Tirman PF et al: A practical approach to imaging of the shoulder with emphasis on MR imaging. Orthop Clin North Am. 28(4): 483-515, 1997
3. Neviaser TJ: The anterior labroligamentous periosteal sleeve avulsion lesion: A cause of anterior instability of the shoulder. Arthroscopy. 9(1): 17-21, 1993

HAGL Lesion

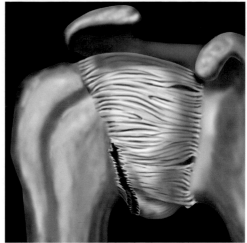

HAGL lesion with humeral avulsion of the glenohumeral ligament. There is tearing of the anterior humeral neck attachment of the IGL.

Key Facts
- **H**umeral **A**vulsion of the inferior **G**lenohumeral **L**igament

Imaging Findings
MR Findings
- Discontinuous capsule at the humeral interface
- Capsule appears "J" shaped on coronal images
- Edema and hemorrhage at humeral interface on axial T2 images
- Hill-Sachs lesion in many cases

Differential Diagnosis
Midcapsular Disruption
- Difficult to exclude in many cases
Extensive Bankart Lesion
- Difficult to asses exact location of capsular disruption in some extensive cases of labral capsular disruption

Pathology
General
- General Path Comments
  o Humeral avulsion of the inferior glenohumeral ligament
- Etiology-Pathogenesis
  o Anterior shoulder dislocation
Gross Pathologic or Surgical Features
- Torn capsule at the humeral interface
- Angled scope is often needed to visualize the defect
Microscopic Features
- Torn glenohumeral capsule with variable amounts of hemorrhage

HAGL Lesion

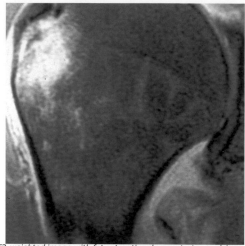

A coronal T2-weighted image with fat saturation demonstrates avulsion of the inferior glenohumeral ligament (axillary pouch) from the humerus resulting in a "J" like appearance of the capsule.

Clinical Issues

Presentation

- Patient with recent anterior shoulder dislocation
- No age predilection
- Recurrent instability in some cases

Treatment & Prognosis

- Conservative treatment in some cases
- Surgical or arthroscopic repair if continued instability

Selected References
1. Stoller DW et al: The Shoulder, in Magnetic Resonance Imaging in Orthopaedics and Sports Medicine. J.B. Lippincott: Philadelphia. 597-742, 1997
2. Tirman PF et al: Humeral avulsion of the anterior shoulder stabilizing structures after anterior shoulder dislocation: Demonstration by MRI and MR arthrography. Skeletal Radiol. 25(8): 743-8, 1996
3. Wolf EM et al: Humeral avulsion of glenohumeral ligaments as a cause of anterior shoulder instability. Arthroscopy. 11(5): 600-7, 1995

Labral Cyst

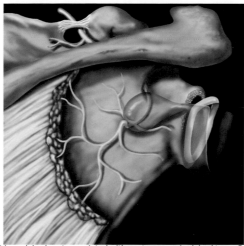

Spinoglenoid paralabral cyst associated with posterosuperior labral tear. Suprascapular nerve entrapment with denervation of the infraspinatus muscle is associated.

Key Facts
- Cyst arises from break in integrity of joint as either a labral tear, degeneration, capsular tear or diverticulum
- May cause suprascapular nerve compression syndrome if located posterosuperiorly
- May cause axillary nerve compression syndrome if located inferiorly and dissects into quadrilateral space
- Associated with instability especially if labral tear remains patent

Imaging Findings
MR Findings
- Cystic-appearing mass arising from or immediately adjacent to labrum or capsule
- May see secondary denervation high signal and/or atrophy of affected muscles if denervation is present
- May see labral tear as high signal extending through labrum on short or long TE sequences

Differential Diagnosis
Neoplasm
- Usually demonstrates internal enhancement
- No association with labral or capsular tear
Muscle Denervation
- From another cause without the presence of the cyst
- Posttraumatic neuropraxis
- Parsonage-Turner syndrome (idiopathic denervation of shoulder girdle muscles)

Labral Cyst

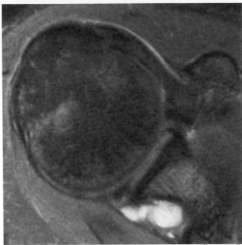

A T2-weighted axial image demonstrates a large cyst extending medially from the posteriorsuperior labrum. The superior labrum was torn (SLAP lesion) giving rise to the cyst. Note the edema in the infraspinatus due to denervation caused by mass effect on the suprascapular nerve.

Pathology
General
- Etiology-Pathogenesis
  - Cyst arises from break in integrity of joint from either a labral tear, degeneration, capsular tear or diverticulum
  - Slow growing typically
  - Tear from which it arises may heal

Gross Pathologic or Surgical Features
- Cyst containing mucoid material
- Often associated with labral tear
- Often associated with denervation of supraspinatus and infraspinatus muscles
- Rarely associated with deltoid and teres minor denervation

Microscopic Features
- Cyst with wall containing spindle-shaped cells
- Cyst contains mucoid material
- Fatty infiltration of muscle tissue in chronically denervated muscles

Clinical Issues
Presentation
- Patient with instability history (labral tear)
- Patient with history suggesting SLAP lesion (superior labral tear)
- Pain and weakness of supraspinatus and infraspinatus and proprioceptive changes (suprascapular denervation)
- Weakness of deltoid and teres minor (axillary denervation)
- Combination of the above

Treatment & Prognosis
- Removal of cyst if symptomatic and repair of labral tear if present

Labral Cyst

Selected References
1. Steiner E et al: Ganglia and cysts around joints. Radiol Clin North Am. 34(2): 395-425, xi-xii, 1996
2. Tirman PF et al: Association of glenoid labral cysts with labral tears and glenohumeral instability: Radiologic findings and clinical significance. Radiology. 190(3): 653-8, 1994
3. Fritz RC et al: Suprascapular nerve entrapment: Evaluation with MR imaging. Radiology. 182(2): 437-44, 1992

Adhesive Capsulitis

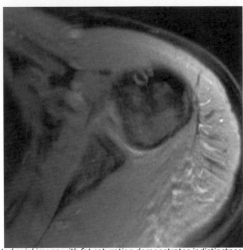

A T2-weighted axial image with fat saturation demonstrates indistinctness and edema of the inferior glenohumeral ligament.

Key Facts
- Inflammation of the inferior shoulder capsule causing limited range of motion and most often a "frozen shoulder"

Imaging Findings
<u>MR Findings</u>
- Indistinct edematous inferior capsule on T2-weighted images most notably coronal and axial
- Thickened capsule measuring greater than 3 mm on coronal images

Differential Diagnosis
<u>Impingement Syndrome</u>
- Adhesive capsulitis results in both passive and active range of motion limitations

Pathology
<u>General</u>
- Etiology-Pathogenesis
  - May be idiopathic or secondary to trauma

<u>Gross Pathologic or Surgical Features</u>
- Thickened indurated inferior capsule

<u>Microscopic Features</u>
- Influx of fibrosis and inflammatory cells

Clinical Issues
<u>Presentation</u>
- Adult patient with painful limited range of motion
- May accompany rotator cuff disease

Adhesive Capsulitis

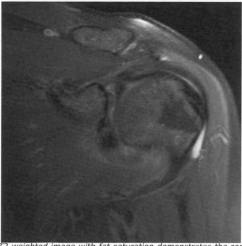

A coronal T2-weighted image with fat saturation demonstrates the same finding.

- Painful and restricted passive and active range of motion at physical examination

<u>Treatment & Prognosis</u>

- Typically physical therapy

Selected References
1. Hannafin JA et al: Adhesive capsulitis. A treatment approach. Clin Orthop. 372:95-109, 2000
2. Carrillon Y et al. Magnetic resonance imaging findings in idiopathic adhesive capsulitis of the shoulder. Rev Rhum Engl Ed. 66(4): 201-6, 1999
3. Warner JJ: Frozen Shoulder: Diagnosis and Management. J Am Acad Orthop Surg. 5(3). 130-40, 1997

Shoulder Osteoarthritis

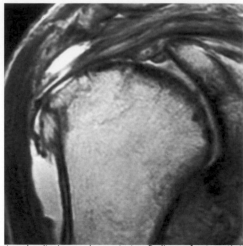

Coronal proton density image demonstrates findings of osteoarthritis including chondromalacia, subcortical sclerosis, osteophyte formation, synovitis, joint effusion.

Key Facts
- Degenerative arthritis characterized by chondromalacia, osteophyte formation, subchondral cysts and synovitis
- Relatively uncommon
- May be found in younger post-operative instability (secondary arthritis)

Imaging Findings
MR Findings
- Cartilage thinning (chondromalacia) seen as diffuse or focal cartilage loss
- Best seen on T2-weighted images with fat saturation
- Subarticular cysts seen as high signal rounded lesions on T2 and gradient echo images
- Osteophyte formation especially involving the humeral head
- Synovitis seen as thickening of the synovium especially on proton density images
- Loose bodies
- May be seen to better advantage on gradient echo images

Plain Film Findings
- Demonstrate findings in more advanced cases

Differential Diagnosis
Inflammatory Arthritis
Synovitis
- Often prominent with erosions that may appear as subarticular cysts
- Other joints often involved

Pathology
General
- Elderly patient
- Younger patient if post-traumatic or post-operative

Shoulder Osteoarthritis

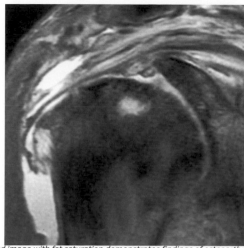

T2-weighted image with fat saturation demonstrates findings of osteoarthritis including chondromalacia, subcortical sclerosis, osteophyte formation, synovitis, joint effusion.

- Relatively uncommon

Gross Pathologic or Surgical Features
- Chondromalacia
- Osteophyte formation
- Subchondral cysts
- Synovitis

Microscopic Features
- Synovial infiltration with PMNs (synovitis)
- Chondromalacia
- Subchondral cysts (geodes)

Clinical Issues

Presentation
- Elderly patient or younger patient if post-traumatic or post-operative
- Insidious onset of pain

Treatment & Prognosis
- Usually conservative
- Total shoulder replacement may be necessary in severe cases

Selected References
1. Kelley M.J. and M.L. Ramsey, Osteoarthritis and traumatic arthritis of the shoulder. J Hand Ther. 13(2): 148-62, 2000
2. Stoller D.W. and E.M. Wolf, The Shoulder, in Magnetic Resonance Imaging in Orthopaedics and Sports Medicine, D.W. Stoller, Editor, J.B. Lippincott: Philadelphia. 597-742. 1997
3. Resnick D., Bone and Joint Imaging. 1 ed. 1989, Philadephia: W.B. Saunders. 1330

Greater Tuberosity Fracture

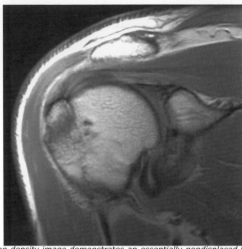

A proton density image demonstrates an essentially nondisplaced fracture.

Key Facts
- Occurs after anterior dislocation of the shoulder or direct impact
- May be x-ray occult

Imaging Findings
Plain Film Findings
- May be occult on plain films

MR Findings
- Increased signal on T2 and decreased signal on T1 images at the fracture site
- Fracture line of decreased signal intensity on MR images

Differential Diagnosis
Rotator Cuff Tear

Subscapularis Rupture

Bankart Lesion
- After anterior dislocation, rotator cuff tear, subscapularis rupture and Bankart lesion can present with posttraumatic pain and decreased range of motion

Pathology
General
- Etiology-Pathogenesis
  - Fracture of greater tuberosity most often after anterior dislocation
  - Occurs in adult population

Gross Pathologic or Surgical Features
- Fracture of greater tuberosity often involving chondral surface grossly
- May be non- or minimally displaced

Microscopic Features
- Disruption of trabeculae and often involving the subchondral endplate and hyaline cartilage with surrounding hemorrhage

Greater Tuberosity Fracture

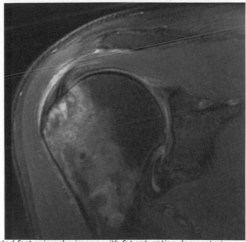

A T2-weighted fast spin echo image with fat saturation demonstrates a nondisplaced fracture. Note the strain of the supraspinatus.

Clinical Issues

Presentation
- Posttraumatic patient most often after anterior dislocation with limited range of motion and pain

Treatment & Prognosis
- Typically conservative unless a large fragment is present with displacement

Selected References
1.   Kim SH et al: Arthroscopic treatment of symptomatic shoulders with minimally displaced greater tuberosity fracture. Arthroscopy. 16(7): 695-700, 2000
2.   Reinus WR et al: Fractures of the greater tuberosity presenting as rotator cuff abnormality: Magnetic resonance demonstration. J Trauma. 44(4): 670-5, 1998
3.   Tirman PF et al: A practical approach to imaging of the shoulder with emphasis on MR imaging. Orthop Clin North Am. 28(4): 483-515, 1997

Internal Impingement

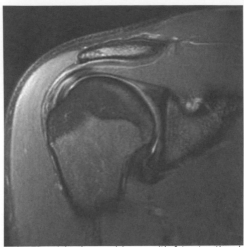

A fast spin echo T2 weighted coronal image with fat saturation demonstrates tendinopathy of the posterior superior rotator cuff (supraspinatus and anterior infraspinatus). These patients were throwing athletes.

Key Facts
- Dynamic compression of the posterior superior aspect of the rotator cuff between the posterosuperior labrum and humeral head
- Usually seen in athletes participating in overhead throwing sports
- Seen in non-athletes who frequently abduct and externally rotate the arm

Imaging Findings
MR Findings
- Undersurface tear of posterior supraspinatus and anterior infraspinatus in early stages, full thickness tear in more advanced cases
- Posterosuperior humeral head chondromalacia and subchondral cystic changes
- Fraying and sometimes tearing of the posterosuperior glenoid labrum
- Abduction and external rotation imaging (ABER) helps define the abnormalities

Differential Diagnosis
Subacromial Impingement
- History is usually suggestive of internal impingement
- Athlete involved in overhead throwing activities
- Instability
- Subluxation while throwing

Pathology
General
- Etiology-Pathogenesis
  - Degeneration and tearing of the supraspinatus and infraspinatus due to shear forces secondary to friction between the posterosuperior rotator cuff, labrum and humeral head during overhead throwing

Internal Impingement

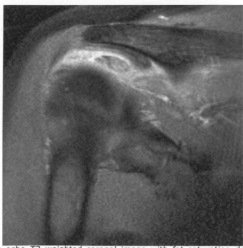

A fast spin echo T2 weighted coronal image with fat saturation demonstrates tendinopathy of the posterior superior rotator cuff (supraspinatus and anterior infraspinatus). These patients were throwing athletes.

Gross Pathologic or Surgical Features
• Tendinosis and tearing of supraspinatus, infraspinatus, labrum and humeral head erosions
• Tendon is indurated, often inflamed and frayed or frankly torn
• Degenerative fraying and/or tearing of the posterosuperior labrum
• Chondromalacia and impaction of the posterosuperior humeral head with varying degrees of subcortical geode formation

Microscopic Features
• Degeneration and varying degrees of inflammatory infiltration of rotator cuff tendons and posterosuperior labrum
• Chondral degeneration and thinning as well as subcortical sclerosis and geode formation of the posterosuperior humeral head

Clinical Issues
Presentation
• Pain with abduction and external rotation in athlete participating in overhead throwing sports
• Adult with occupational activities including abduction external rotation activities
• Varying degrees of both rotator cuff and instability physical examination signs

Treatment & Prognosis
• Physical therapy
• Arthroscopic debridement of rotator cuff and labral fraying
• Repair of rotator cuff tear

Selected References
1. Tirman PF et al: Posterosuperior glenoid impingement of the shoulder: Findings at MR imaging and MR arthrography with arthroscopic correlation. Radiology. 193(2): 431-6, 1994
2. Jobe CM: Evidence for a superior glenoid impingement upon the rotator cuff. J Shoulder Elbow Surg. 2(part 2): S19, 1993

3.   Walch GP et al: Impingement of the deep surface of the supraspinatus tendon on the posterosuperior glenoid rim: An arthroscopic study. J Shoulder Elbow. 1:238-45, 1992

Anterosuperior Variations

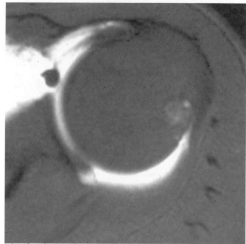

Axial T1-weighted arthrographic image with fat saturation demonstrates absence of the anterior superior labrum associated with a cord-like middle glenohumeral ligament.

Key Facts
- Detached anterior superior labrum from the mid glenoid notch to the biceps anchor: sublabral hole
- Absent anterior superior labrum in combination with a "cord-like" middle glenohumeral ligament: Buford complex

Imaging Findings
MR Findings
- Detached but otherwise normal-appearing anterior-superior labrum from the mid glenoid notch to the biceps anchor–sublabral hole
- Absent anterior-superior labrum in combination with a "cord-like" middle glenohumeral ligament: Buford complex

Differential Diagnosis
Torn Anterosuperior Labrum
- Labrum is usually irregular and of high signal
- History may be helpful

Pathology
General
- Normal anatomic variations
Gross Pathologic or Surgical Features
- Detached or absent anterosuperior labrum from mid-glenoid notch to biceps anchor
Microscopic Features
- No abnormalities

Clinical Presentation
- Not symptomatic
Treatment & Prognosis
- None necessary

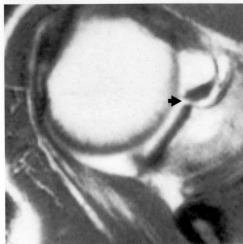

Axial T1-weighted arthrographic image through the anterior superior joint demonstrates normal detachment of the anterior superior labrum (arrow) in a sublabral foramen.

Selected References
1. Beltran JJ et al: MR arthrography of the shoulder: Variants and pitfalls. Radiographics. 17(6): 1403-12, 1997
2. Stoller DW. MR arthrography of the glenohumeral joint. Radiol Clin North Am. 35(1): 97-116, 1997
3. Williams MM et al: The Buford complex-the "cord-like" middle glenohumeral ligament and absent anterosuperior complex: A normal anatomic capsulolabral variant. Arthroscopy. 10(3): 241-7, 1994

PocketRadiologist™
Musculoskeletal
100 Top Diagnoses

ELBOW

Lateral Epicondylitis

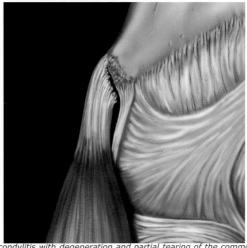

Lateral epicondylitis with degeneration and partial tearing of the common extensor tendon.

Key Facts
- Degeneration of the common extensor tendon secondary to overload caused by chronic varus stress
- Also known as tennis elbow

Imaging Findings
MR Findings
- Increased signal intensity within the common extensor tendon origin at the lateral epicondyle, tendon is often thickened
- Fluid signal intensity within the tendon in the case of a partial tear or complete tears
- Fast spin echo T2-weighted images with fat sat or STIR images demonstrate the increased signal to best advantage
- Increase signal intensity within the common extensor muscle belly in the case of muscle strain
- Strains and tears of the lateral ulnar collateral ligament in advanced cases
- Osteochondral injuries of the humeral trochlea
- Increased signal in trochlea on T2-weighted images
- May see chondromalacia and underlying bone marrow edema or cysts
- Loose bodies may be present

Differential Diagnosis
Trauma and Fibrosis of the Radiohumeral Meniscus
- MRI can define the normal tendon
  - Loose bodies

Pathology
General
- Etiology-Pathogenesis
  - Overuse syndrome caused by chronic varus stress across the elbow

Lateral Epicondylitis

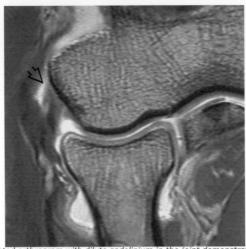

A T1-weighted arthrogram with dilute gadolinium in the joint demonstrates a tear of the common extensor tendon origin from the lateral epicondyle (arrow).

- o   Adults
- o   Most common reason for visit to the doctor's office for elbow pain

Gross Pathologic or Surgical Features
- Thickening of the tendon, +/- macroscopic partial tearing or through-and-through tearing
- May include tear of the lateral ulnar collateral ligament

Microscopic Features
- Angiofibroblastic tendinosis +/- inflammation

Clinical Issues
Presentation
- Adult patient with lateral elbow pain
- Tennis player or other activity resulting in chronic, repeated varus stress less common than athlete

Treatment & Prognosis
- Physical therapy and steroid injection with decrease in physical activity
- Tendon release
- Tendon repair

Selected References
1.   Ciccotti MG: Epicondylitis in the athlete. Instr Course Lect. 48:375-81, 1999
2.   Fritz RC et al: The Elbow, in Magnetic Resonance Imaging in Orthopedica and Sports Medicine, D.W. Stoller, Editor. J.B. Lippincott: Philadelphia. 743-849, 1997
3.   Jobe FW et al: Lateral and Medial Epicondylitis of the Elbow. J Am Acad Orthop Surg. 2(1):1-8, 1994

Medial Epicondylitis

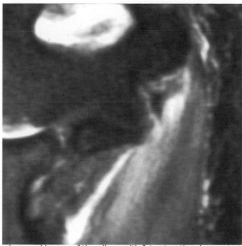

A T2 weighted coronal image of the elbow with fat saturation demonstrates increased signal intensity within the flexor pronator muscle belly indicating a strain.

Key Facts
- Degeneration of the common flexor tendon secondary to overload caused by chronic valgus stress
- Also known as golfer's elbow, pitcher's elbow

Imaging Findings
MR Findings
- Medial tension overload
  - Increased signal intensity within the common flexor tendon origin at the medial epicondyle, tendon often thickened
- Fluid signal intensity within the tendon in the case of a partial tear or complete tears
  - Fast spin echo T2-weighted images with fat sat or STIR images demonstrate the increased signal to best advantage
  - Increase signal intensity within the common flexor muscle belly in the case of muscle strain
  - Avulsion of medial epicondyle in skeletally immature individuals
  - Strains and tears of the ulnar collateral ligament
  - Ulnar neuritis
    - High signal and thickening of the nerve usually within the cubital tunnel
- Lateral compression
  - Osteochondral injuries of the humeral capitellum
    - Increased signal in capitellum on T2-weighted images
    - May see chondromalacia and underlying bone marrow edema or cysts
    - Loose bodies may be present

Differential Diagnosis
Ulnar Collateral Ligament Strain Without Tendon Disruption
- Coronal T2 images useful to distinguish between the two

Medial Epicondylitis

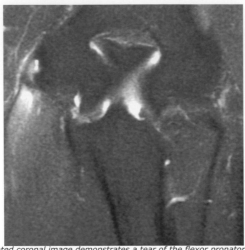

A T2 weighted coronal image demonstrates a tear of the flexor pronator origin from the medial epicondyle.

Pathology
General
* Etiology-Pathogenesis
  * Overuse syndrome found in athletes participating in throwing sports
  * Due to repeated valgus stress causing tendon degeneration
  * Children and adults
    * In children the injury is often to the medial epicondyle itself manifesting as a stress fracture or avulsion of the epicondyle

Gross Pathologic or Surgical Features
* Thickening of the tendon, +/- macroscopic partial tearing or through-and-through tearing
* Avulsed epicondyle in the case of some children
* May include tear of the ulnar collateral ligament

Microscopic Features
* Microscopic tendon degeneration with macroscopic partial or complete tear surrounded by hemorrhage and inflammation

Clinical Issues
Presentation
* Athlete participating in throwing sports with onset of medial elbow pain

Treatment & Prognosis
* Physical therapy and steroid injection with decrease in physical activity
* Tendon release
* Tendon repair

Selected References
1. Chen FS et al: Medial elbow problems in the overhead-throwing athlete. J Am Acad Orthop Surg. 9(2):99-113, 2001
2. Fritz RC: MR imaging of sports injuries of the elbow. Magn Reson Imaging Clin N Am, 7(1):51-72, viii, 1999
3. Ciccotti MG: Epicondylitis in the athlete. Instr Course Lect. 48:375-81, 1999

MCL Injury (Elbow)

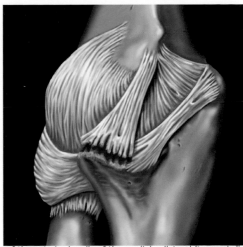

Tear of the anterior bundle of the medial collateral ligament distally.

Key Facts
- Degeneration and tearing of the MCL caused by repetitive valgus stress in athletes during the acceleration phase of throwing or as acute valgus injury
- Anterior band is most important structure injured

Imaging Findings
MR Findings
- Increased signal on T2-weighted images with fat saturation or STIR images within the ligament, most commonly the anterior band
- Discontinuity of ligament fibers
- Increased signal (stress response or fracture) at humeral origin site or attachment site on the ulnar coronoid
- Arthrography demonstrates "T" sign (contrast interposed between the partially torn ligament and the medial aspect of the coronoid forming the letter "T" on its side) in cases of distal partial tears that spare the superficial fibers
- Extravasation of contrast in cases of complete ruptures
- Heterotopic ossification or epicondylar avulsion seen as increased signal (fat in bone marrow), corticated structure on T1 and proton density images

Differential Diagnosis
Medial Epicondylitis with Intact MCL
- MRI can differentiate between these two entities

Pathology
General
- Etiology-Pathogenesis
  - Acute in valgus stress injury
  - Children (usually athletes) or adults

MCL Injury (Elbow)

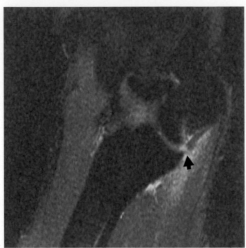

A STIR coronal image in a baseball player demonstrates a rupture of the distal ulnar collateral ligament (arrow) associated with a strain of the flexor pronator muscle belly.

- o Midsubstance ruptures most common followed by distal then proximal ruptures

Gross Pathologic or Surgical Features
- • Thickened, partially torn or completely torn anterior band of the ulnar collateral ligament

Microscopic Features
- • Degeneration, partial or complete rupture
- • Variable amounts of hemorrhage and inflammatory cells

Staging or Grading Criteria
- • Partial tear
  - o Proximal
  - o Mid substance
  - o Distal
- • Complete tear

Clinical Issues

Presentation
- • Patient after valgus stress injury
  - o Usually acute episode superimposed on chronic repetitive valgus stress
- • Child (usually athlete) or adult

Treatment & Prognosis
- • Consecutive management in an athlete
- • Repair of complete disruption in athletes

Selected References
1. Chen FS et al: Medial elbow problems in the overhead-throwing athlete. J Am Acad Orthop Surg. 9(2):99-113, 2001
2. Fritz RC: MR imaging of sports injuries of the elbow. Magn Reson Imaging Clin N Am. 7(1):51-72, viii, 1999
3. Schwartz ML, et al: Ulnar collateral ligament injury in the throwing athlete: Evaluation with saline-enhanced MR arthrography. Radiology. 197(1):297-9, 1995

Elbow Instability

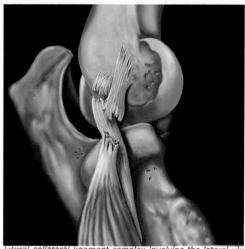

Tear of the lateral collateral ligament complex involving the lateral ulnar collateral ligament and tear of the common extensor tendon. This represents a case of posterolateral rotatory instability.

Key Facts
- Three stages of progressive instability beginning with subluxation and progressing to dislocation
- Essential lesion is a tear of the lateral ulnar collateral ligament (LUCL)

Imaging Findings
MR Findings
- Tear of lateral ulnar collateral ligament (LUCL) at origin on the humerus
- Disruption of ligamentous fibers with fluid signal intensity on T2-weighted images
- May be associated with lateral epicondylitis (tendinosis and or tearing of the common extensor tendon origin)
- Perched elbow is coronoid perched on dorsal aspect of trochlea and disruption of anterior and posterior capsule with high signal intensity (edema) around the injury
- Dislocation involves all of the above plus complete dislocation of the radius and ulna and progressive disruption of the medial collateral ligament

Plain Film Findings
- Plain films may show dislocation or perched elbow or they may be normal if spontaneous reduction has occurred

Differential Diagnosis
Lateral Epicondylitis
- May mimic posterolateral rotatory instability (PLRI)
- Advanced cases may include disruption of the LUCL so overlapping signs may develop

Clinically Swollen Tender Elbow
- From a variety of causes (most often posttraumatic)
- PLRI may be a diagnosis of exclusion

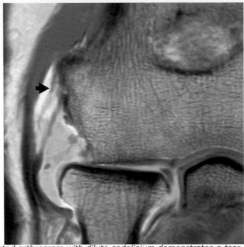

A T1-weighted arthrogram with dilute gadolinium demonstrates a tear of the origin of the lateral ulnar collateral ligament and disruption of the lateral capsule and extensor tendon (arrow).

- MRI very helpful in these cases

Pathology
General
- Etiology-Pathogenesis
    o Relatively uncommon abnormalities
    o Most often develops insidiously after initial injury
    o Recurrent complete dislocation occurs more frequently in children
Gross Pathologic or Surgical Features
- Tear of origin of LUCL with or without lateral epicondylitis for PLRI
- Dislocated ulna and radius for more advanced stages
Microscopic Features
- Microscopic and macroscopic tearing of the LUCL (early on) followed by the anterior and posterior elbow joint capsule and then medial ligamentous structures
- Variable amounts of hemorrhage and inflammatory cells
Staging or Grading Criteria
- Stage I
    o PLRI: Posterolateral subluxation of the ulna and radius relative to the humerus due to a tear of the lateral ulnar collateral ligament
- Stage II
    o Perched elbow: Coronoid perched on trochlea
- Stage III A
    o Complete dislocation with tear of the posterior band of the ulnar (medial) collateral ligament
    o Elbow is stable to valgus stress
- Stage III B
    o Complete dislocation with tear of the entire ulnar (medial) collateral ligament
    o Elbow is unstable in all directions

Elbow Instability

Clinical Issues

Presentation
- Swelling and pain after traumatic event
- Patient is often guarding leading to difficult presentation
- Positive elbow pivot shift test
- Supination/valgus added during flexion causing the radius and ulna to sublux posteriorly

Treatment & Prognosis
- Repair of ligament in patients with symptomatic instability

Selected References
1. O'Driscoll SW: Elbow instability. Acta Orthop Belg. 65(4):404-15, 1999
2. Bredella MA et al: MR imaging findings of lateral ulnar collateral ligament abnormalities in patients with lateral epicondylitis. AJR. 173(5):1379-82, 1999
3. Potter HG et al: Posterolateral rotatory instability of the elbow: Usefulness of MR imaging in diagnosis. Radiology. 204(1):185-9, 1997

Ulnar Neuritis

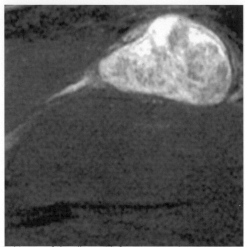

A T2-weighted image of the elbow with fat saturation demonstrates an ulnar nerve neuroma as a cause of this patient's ulnar neuritis.

Key Facts
- Compression of the ulnar nerve usually within the cubital tunnel
- Most commonly caused by a thickened cubital tunnel retinaculum resulting in dynamic compression during flexion
- Can be caused by any mass compression of the nerve or as the result of a posttraumatic neuropraxis

Imaging Findings
MR Findings
- Displacement or flattening of the nerve
- Thickened cubital tunnel retinaculum
- Mass lesion with proximal swelling of the nerve seen best on T2-weighted fat saturated images
- Increased signal intensity of the nerve itself

Differential Diagnosis
Enlarged Perineural Veins
- Often contain flow void
Increased Signal Intensity Nerve in Normal Cases
- Pathologic nerve is of greater increased signal intensity on T2-weighted (especially fat saturated) images and is variably thickened
Brachial Plexitis
- Other nerves most often involved

Pathology
General
- Etiology-Pathogenesis
  - Most commonly seen in adults
  - Ulnar neuropraxis often secondary to repeated valgus stress injury and medial epicondylitis

Ulnar Neuritis

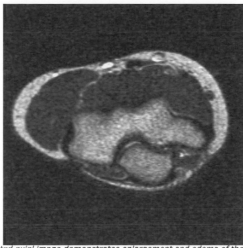

A T2-weighted axial image demonstrates enlargement and edema of the ulnar nerve secondary to medial epicondylitis.

- Epidemiology
  - 22% of population suffers from dynamic compression during flexion in association with a thickened cubital tunnel retinaculum
  - 10% of population suffers from static compression in association with an anomalous muscle, the anconeus epitrochlearis

Gross Pathologic or Surgical Features
- Edematous/ indurated nerve often surrounded by fibrous stranding
- Heterotopic ossification or other mass may be found compressing the nerve
- Anconeus epitrochlearis may be found in place of the cubital tunnel retinaculum

Microscopic Features
- Edematous nerve with variable numbers of inflammatory cells

Clinical Issues

Presentation
- Adult or child with pain and paresthesias in forearm in the ulnar nerve distribution
- Athletes with medial epicondylitis and pain and paresthesias in the ulnar nerve distribution

Treatment & Prognosis
- Physical therapy
- Removal of osteophyte or anconeous if paresthesias present

Selected References
1. Chen FS et al: Medial elbow problems in the overhead-throwing athlete. J Am Acad Orthop Surg. 9(2):99-113, 2001
2. Fritz RC: MR imaging of sports injuries of the elbow. Magn Reson Imaging Clin N Am. 7(1):51-72, viii, 1999
3. Ciccotti MG: Medial collateral ligament instability and ulnar neuritis in the athlete's elbow. Instr Course Lect. 48:383-91, 1999

Biceps Tendon Rupture

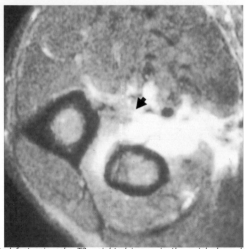

Fat saturated fast spin echo T2-weighted image in the axial plane demonstrates complete rupture of the biceps tendon (arrow) with surrounding hemorrhage.

Key Facts
- Rupture of distal biceps tendon from the insertion site on the radial tuberosity
- Eccentric contraction against resistance such as sudden forced extension of a flexed forearm

Imaging Findings
MR Findings
- Usually complete disruption from the radial tuberosity with variable degrees of retraction seen on all imaging sequences as discontinuous decreased signal intensity tendon
- Increased signal intensity fluid surrounds the tendon and is best visualized on fat saturated fast spin echo T2-weighted or STIR images
- Partial tears seen as fluid within but not completely through the tendon are uncommon
- Tendinosis is seen as increased signal intensity within a variably thickened tendon

Plain Film Findings
- Hypertrophy of the radial tuberosity can be seen on plain films

Differential Diagnosis
Bicipital Radial Bursitis
- Fluid within the bursae of the antecubital fossa
- Intact biceps tendon seen on MRI

Pathology
General
- Etiology-Pathogenesis
  - Occurs almost exclusively in adult men, dominant arm, suffered forced extension of a flexed forearm
  - Average age = 55 years

Biceps Tendon Rupture

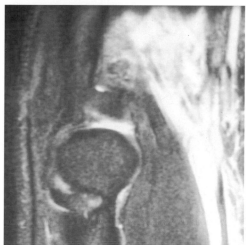

Fat saturated fast spin echo T2-weighted image in the sagittal plane demonstrates complete rupture of the biceps tendon with surrounding hemorrhage.

o   Body builders/weight lifters may present earlier

Gross Pathologic or Surgical Features
- Disrupted tendon with variable degrees of retraction
- Hypertrophic bicipital radial bursitis may be present

Microscopic Features
- Tendinosis and macroscopic tear of the tendon with variable amounts of hemorrhage and inflammatory cells

Clinical Issues

Presentation
- Typically a middle-aged man who suffered forced extension of a flexed forearm
- Biceps muscle belly "balls up" in proximal forearm giving "popeye" sign
- May not be retracted to a great degree if aponeurosis is intact
- Aponeurosis is the lacertus fibrosis that extends from the myotendinous junction to the medial deep fascia of the forearm

Treatment & Prognosis
- Surgical repair

Selected References
1. Bell RH et al: Repair of distal biceps brachii tendon ruptures. J Shoulder Elbow Surg. 9(3):223-6, 2000
2. Fritz RC: MR imaging of sports injuries of the elbow. Magn Reson Imaging Clin N Am. 7(1):51-72, viii, 1999
3. Le Huec JC et al: Distal rupture of the tendon of biceps brachii. Evaluation by MRI and the results of repair. J Bone Joint Surg Br. 78(5):767-70, 1996

Bicipital Radial Bursitis

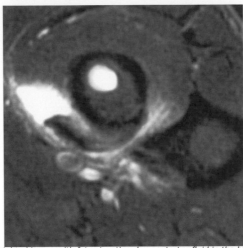

Axial T2 weighted image with fat saturation demonstrates fluid in the bicipital radial bursa.

Key Facts
- Inflammation of the bicipital radial bursa
- Bursa located between the distal biceps tendon and the anterior aspect of the radial tuberosity
- May fill with fluid and present as mass on antecubital fossa

Imaging Findings
General Features
- High signal, fluid intensity mass interposed between the distal biceps tendon and the anterior aspect of the radial tuberosity
- May demonstrate thin rim enhancement after gadolinium administration
- Variable amounts of internal debris

Differential Diagnosis
Biceps Tendinosis or Partial Tear
- See tendinopathy on MR images
- May be seen together

Pathology
General
- Etiology-Pathogenesis
  - Inflammation of the bursa with variable amounts of fluid within it
  - Typically adult patient
  - Associated with biceps tendinopathy
Gross Pathologic or Surgical Features
- Indurated, fluid filled bursa of variable size
Microscopic Features
- Hypertrophied bursal synovial lining with infiltration of inflammatory cells
- Fibrosis and granulation tissue often present

Bicipital Radial Bursitis

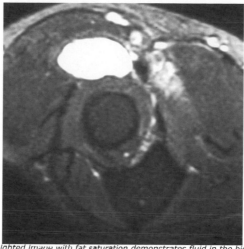

Axial T2 weighted image with fat saturation demonstrates fluid in the bicipital radial bursa.

Clinical Issues

Presentation
- Antecubital mass (if large) or pain often associated with supination
- Patient may have history of biceps pain

Treatment & Prognosis
- Conservation management typically
- Extensive cases require bursectomy

Selected References
1. Ramsey ML: Distal biceps tendon injuries: Diagnosis and management. J Am Acad Orthop Surg. 7(3):199-207, 1999
2. Fritz RC et al: MR imaging of the elbow. An update. Radiol Clin North Am. 35(1):117-44, 1997
3. Fritz RC et al: The Elbow, in Magnetic Resonance Imaging in Orthopedica and Sports Medicine. D.W. Stoller, Editor. J.B. Lippincott: Philadelphia. 743-849, 1997

Olecranon Bursitis

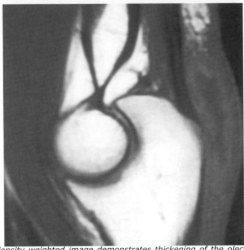

A proton density weighted image demonstrates thickening of the olecranon bursa and an effusion.

Key Facts
- Inflammation of the olecranon bursa
- Bursa located between integument and olecranon process and triceps insertion within the subcutaneous adipose tissue
- Miner's or student's elbow

Imaging Findings
MR Findings
- High-signal, fluid intensity mass in superficial soft tissues adjacent to the olecranon process and triceps insertion
- May demonstrate a thin rim enhancement after gadolinium administration
- Variable amounts of internal, typically hemorrhagic debris
- Rarely osteomyelitis is present

Plain Film Findings
- May see swelling and /or air on plain films
- May see olecranon spur in chronic bursitis

Differential Diagnosis
Triceps Tendinosis or Partial Tear
- See tendinopathy on MR images
- May be seen together

Solid Mass
- Enhancement may help as uncomplicated bursitis will demonstrate only rim enhancement
- Chronic florid bursitis may demonstrate diffuse enhancement

Pathology
General
- Etiology-Pathogenesis
  - Inflammation of the bursa with variable amounts of fluid within it

Olecranon Bursitis

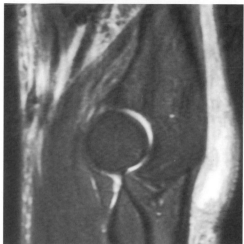

A fast spin echo T2 weighted image demonstrates thickening of the olecranon bursa and an effusion.

o   Adolescent or adult patient
o   Associated with triceps tendinopathy and tears
o   Secondary to acute or repetitive trauma
o   Traumatic bursitis commonly a football injury associated with artificial turf
o   May be secondary to systemic disease

Gross Pathologic or Surgical Features
•   Indurated, fluid-filled bursa of variable size

Microscopic Features
•   Hypertrophied bursal synovial lining with infiltration of inflammatory cells
•   Fibrosis
•   Nodules of granulation tissues often present
•   May be infected and most commonly due to staphylococcus aureus
    o   Usually posttraumatic

Clinical Issues

Presentation
•   Swelling and pain secondary to acute or repetitive trauma to the area of the olecranon process
•   May be seen in patients with underlying systemic disease

Treatment & Prognosis
•   Conservative treatment unless extensive
•   Extensive cases require bursectomy

Selected References
1.   Fritz RC et al: The Elbow, in Magnetic Resonance Imaging in Orthopedica and Sports Medicine, D.W. Stoller, Editor. J.B. Lippincott: Philadelphia. 743-849, 1997
2.   Fritz RC et al: MR imaging of the elbow. An update. Radiol Clin North Am. 35(1):117-44, 1997
3.   Steiner E et al: Ganglia and cysts around joints. Radiol Clin North Am. 34(2):395-425, xi-xii, 1996

Triceps Tendon Rupture

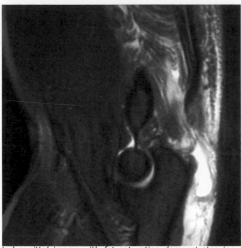

A T2-weighted sagittal image with fat saturation demonstrates increased signal intensity within the distal triceps tendon consistent with a partial tear.

Key Facts
- Rupture of triceps tendon from the insertion site on the olecranon
- Eccentric contraction against resistance such as sudden forced flexion of an extended forearm or direct trauma onto the tendon with the muscle contracted and the forearm extended

Imaging Findings
General Features
- A tear or gap in the tendon which can become filled with joint or bursal fluid or granulation tissue

MR Findings
- Partial or complete disruption from the olecranon with variable degrees of retraction seen on all imaging sequences as a discontinuous decreased signal intensity tendon usually with a fluid (increased) signal intensity gap
- Increased signal intensity fluid surrounds the tendon and is best visualized on fat saturated fast spin echo T2-weighted or STIR images
- Partial tears seen as fluid within but not completely through the tendon are uncommon
- Tendinosis is seen as increased signal intensity within a variably thickened tendon

Differential Diagnosis
Olecranon Bursitis Clinically
- Most common in adult men, dominant arm
- Uncommon injury
- May occur in setting of sports

Pathology
General
- Etiology-Pathogenesis

Triceps Tendon Rupture

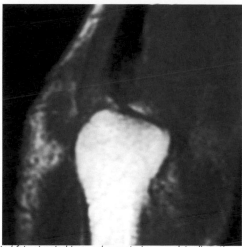

A T2-weighted fat saturated image demonstrates complete disruption of the triceps tendon.

- ○ Eccentric contraction against resistance such as sudden forced flexion of an extended forearm or direct trauma onto the tendon with the muscle contracted and the forearm extended

Gross Pathologic or Surgical Features
- Usually thickened indurated tendon edges
- Break in integrity of tendon
- Disrupted tendon with variable degrees of retraction

Microscopic Features
- Break in integrity of tendon
- Preexisting collagen degeneration without significant influx of inflammatory cells: "Tendinosis" is preferred term over tendinitis
- Fatty infiltration of muscle tissue in chronically torn tendons
- Tendinosis and macroscopic tear of the tendon with variable amounts of hemorrhage and inflammatory cells

Clinical Issues

Presentation
- Typically a middle-aged man who suffered forced flexion of an extended forearm
- Increased incidence in patients who have undergone a previous olecranon bursectomy

Treatment & Prognosis
- Repair

Selected References
1. Dev S et al: Rupture of the triceps muscle at its attachments. Injury. 30(1):70-1, 1999
2. Strauch RJ: Biceps and triceps injuries of the elbow. Orthop Clin North Am. 30(1):95-107, 1999
3. Fritz R.C. and D.W. Stoller, The Elbow, in Magnetic Resonance Imaging in Orthopedica and Sports Medicine, D.W. Stoller, Editor. J.B. Lippincott: Philadelphia. 743-849, 1997

Capitellar Osteochondritis

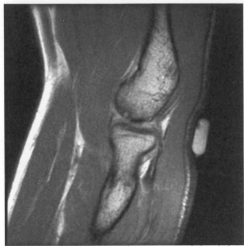

A proton density weighted sagittal image demonstrates subchondral erosions of the capitellum.

Key Facts
- Necrosis of bone followed by healing response and reossification
- Capitellum is most common site in the elbow
- Chronic valgus stress with lateral impaction seen in gymnasts and adolescent pitchers

Imaging Findings
MR Findings
- Decreased or intermediate signal intensity within the capitellum in contrast to normal increased signal intensity marrow
- Loose osteochondritic fragment may be seen
- Fluid between interface of fragment and donor site in capitellum in unstable lesions
- Cyst-like lesions in capitellum underneath the fragment in unstable lesions

Differential Diagnosis
Panner's Disease
- Seen in younger patients (5-11 year old patients)
- Loose body formation and residual deformity usually not seen in Panner's disease
- Probably avascular necrosis secondary to trauma
Pseudodefect of the Capitellum
Normal Anatomy
Posteriorly Located

Pathology
General
- Lesion of adolescence often seen in athletes
- Loose body formation and residual deformity often present

Capitellar Osteochondritis

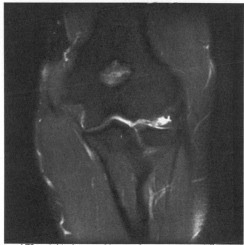

A fat suppressed T2-weighted coronal image demonstrates subchondral erosion with fluid signal intensity.

Gross Pathologic or Surgical Features
- Necrotic desiccated bone fragment in unstable lesions

Microscopic Features
- Osteonecrosis with variable amounts of healing

Staging or Grading Criteria
- Stable lesions
  - Small size
  - No fluid between interface of humerus and osteochondritic fragment
- Unstable lesions
- Large size (typically greater than a centimeter)
- Cyst-like lesion beneath the osteochondrotic lesion
- Contains loose granulation tissue
- Loose fragment
- Fluid insinuating beneath the fragment at arthrography

Clinical Issues
Presentation
- 13-16 year children, often athletes with insidious onset of pain or history of trauma

Treatment & Prognosis
- Stable lesions treated with rest and splinting
- Unstable lesions often treated with abrasion chondroplasty or microfracture unless large, displaced fragment is found

Selected References
1. Kaeding CC: Musculoskeletal injuries in adolescents. Prim Care. 25(1):211-23, 1998
2. Field LD et al. Common elbow injuries in sport. Sports Med. 26(3):193-205, 1999
3. Fritz RC: MR imaging of osteochondral and articular lesions. Magn Reson Imaging Clin N Am. 5(3):579-602, 1997

WRIST AND HAND

Scapholunate Ligament Tear

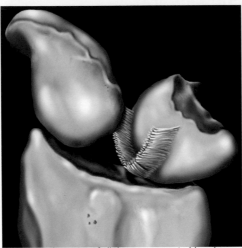

Scapholunate ligament disruption of all three components (dorsal, membranous and volar).

Key Facts
- Dissociation between scaphoid and lunate
- Scaphoid becomes flexed relative to lunate
- Scapholunate (SL) angle increases to more than 70 degrees
- SL ligament made up of dorsal, membranous and volar fibers

Imaging Findings
MR Findings
- Discrete linear signal in partial or complete tear
- Complete ligamentous disruption
- Synovial fluid communication between radiocarpal and midcarpal compartment
- Degenerative perforations occur in thin membranous portion (dorsal and volar fibers are intact)
- MR arthrography may assist in identifying flap tears, perforations and the integrity of the dorsal component

Imaging Recommendations
- Recommend fat-suppressed T2-weighted FSE sequence (coronal plane)

Differential Diagnosis
SL Ligament Sprain
- Ligament fibers are still in continuity

Pathology
General
- General Path Comments
  - Scaphoid attachment of the SL ligament has less Sharpey's fibers than the lunate attachment (more susceptible to tear)
  - Dorsal component is oriented transversely: Forms a thick bundle important in maintaining stability and thus less likely to tear

Scapholunate Ligament Tear

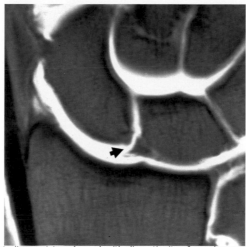

Scapholunate ligament tear (arrow) with discontinuity of membranous component at scaphoid attachment (FST1 MR arthrogram).

- ○ Occult ganglions may be associated with partial tear of the dorsal fibers
- ○ Membranous component is triangular shaped and attached to articular cartilage and bone
- ○ Dorsal and volar fibers attached directly to bone
- • Etiology-Pathogenesis
  - ○ Excessive loading to dorsal capsule with trauma

Clinical Issues
Presentation
- • Associated with a scaphoid avulsion fracture
- • Seen in DISI (dorsal intercalated segment instability)

Treatment & Prognosis
- • Debride membranous tears
- • Open suture repair of torn ligament plus immobilization
- • Ligament rupture plus rotatory subluxation requires intercarpal fusion or dorsal capsulodesis

Selected References
1. Brown RR et al: Extrinsic and intrinsic ligaments of the wrist: normal and pathologic anatomy at MR arthrography with three-compartment enhancement. Radiographics. 18:667-74, 1998
2. Totterman SM et al: Scapholunate ligament: normal MR appearance on three-dimensional gradient-recalled-echo images. Radiology. 200:241-337, 1996
3. Timins ME et al: MR imaging of the major carpal stabilizing ligaments: normal anatomy and clinical examples. Radiographics. 25:575-87, 1995

Lunotriquetral Ligament Tear

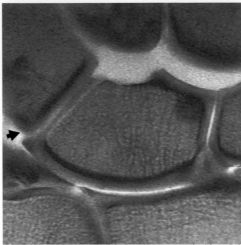

Flap tear (arrow) of lunotriquetral (LT) ligament associated with radial TFC tear. A medial lunate facet with distal lunate chondromalacia is also demonstrated (coronal T1-weighted MR arthrogram).

Key Facts
- Dissociation between triquetrum and lunate
- Volar flexion of lunate
- Lunotriquetral (LT) ligament made up of dorsal, membranous and volar fibers

Imaging Findings
MR Findings
- Absence of horseshoe-shaped structure
- Insertional site tear or perforations appreciated on MR arthrography
- More difficult to separate components of volar, dorsal and membranous fibers without MR arthrography technique
- Normal LT ligament does not extend into LT joint
- Delta-shaped or linear ligament is appreciated on coronal images
- Insertional tear or perforation may require MR arthrography
Imaging Recommendations
- Recommend fat suppressed (FS) T2-weighted FSE sequence (coronal plane)

Differential Diagnosis
LT Ligament Sprain
- No extension of fluid across LT fibers or discontinuity of ligament

Pathology
General
- General Path Comments
  - Normal LT ligament may appear more lax
  - Volar and dorsal portions of LT ligament attached directly to bone
  - Membranous portion attaches to hyaline articular cartilage
  - Volar component is stronger than dorsal component

Lunotriquetral Ligament Tear

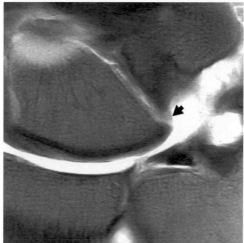

Tear (arrow) of the volar component of the LT ligament. TFC tear and proximal lunate chondral degeneration are shown (coronal T1-weighted MR arthrogram).

- o Membranous component is weakest and may show communication of fluid across interval
- o Scapholunate (SL) angle is decreased to less than 30 degrees
- o Capitolunate (CL) angle may measure up to 30 degrees
- o VISI (volar intercalated segment instability) pattern requires disruption of both LT intrinsic and dorsal extrinsic ligaments
- Etiology-Pathogenesis
  - o Degenerative versus ulnar sided trauma on outstretched hand

Clinical Issues

Presentation
- Associated VISI pattern
- Ulnar shortening if no VISI but positive ulnar variance present

Treatment & Prognosis
- Torn LT ligament repaired
- LT intercarpal fusion also used to treat LT ligament tear
- Nonunion may complicate LT fusion
- New techniques: Bone grafts and compression fixation devices

Selected References
1. Smith DK: MR imaging of normal and injured wrist ligaments. MRI Clinics of North America Philadelphia. 3:229, 1995
2. Smith DK et al: Lunotriquetral interosseous ligament of the wrist. MR appearances in asymptomatic volunteers and arthrographically normal wrists. Radiology. 191:199, 1994
3. Rominger MB et al: MR imaging of anatomy and tears of wrist ligaments. Radiographics. 13.1233, 1993

Ulnolunate Abutment

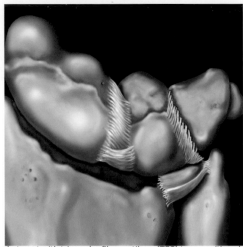

Ulnolunate abutment with triangular fibrocartilage (TFC) tear, positive ulnar variance, lunotriquetral ligament tear and subchondral degeneration of the proximal lunate and triquetrum.

Key Facts
- Equivalent terms: Ulnar impaction syndrome, ulnocarpal abutment and ulnolunate impaction syndrome
- Associated with positive ulnar variance
- TFC tears in chondral lesions of lunate and lunotriquetral (LT) ligament tears

Imaging Findings
Plain Film Findings
- Positive ulnar variance on conventional radiographs

Scintigraphy Findings
- Nonspecific uptake ulnolunate region on bone scintigraphy

CT Findings
- Sclerosis proximal ulnar aspect lunate and proximal radial aspect triquetrum with or without subchondral cystic changes

MR Findings
- Central perforation of TFC
- Neutral or positive ulnar variance
- Eccentric sclerosis proximal ulnar aspect lunate and proximal radial aspect of triquetrum
- +/- cystic change
- Sclerosis hypointense on T1 and T2-weighted images
- Cystic degeneration intermediate to hyperintense on T2-weighted images
- Chondromalacia distal ulna
- Hyperintense fluid across torn LT ligament on T2 (FST2-FSE) images

Ulnolunate Abutment

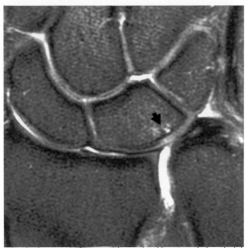

Early findings in ulnolunate abutment with proximal lunate subchondral degeneration, (arrow) TFC tear and LT ligament tear. Note positive ulnar variance (FST2-FSE coronal MR image).

Differential Diagnosis
Kienböck's Disease
- Sclerosis associated with the ischemic change is central and not eccentric
- Negative ulnar variance associated

Pathology
General
- Etiology-Pathogenesis
  - Compression of distal ulna on medial surface of lunate
  - Ulnar styloid fractures contribute to impaction between ulnar styloid segment and proximal lunate
  - Rheumatoid arthritis associated with excessive ulnar length

Clinical Issues
Presentation
- Painful compression between distal ulna and lunate
Treatment & Prognosis
- TFCC debridement and ulnar shortening

Selected References
1. Escobedo EM et al: MR imaging of ulnar impaction. Skel Radiol. 24:85, 1995
2. Schurman AH et al: The ulno-carpal abutment syndrome. Follow-up of the water procedure J Hand Surg [Br]. 20:171, 1995
3. Friedman SL et al: The ulnar impaction syndrome. Hand Clin. 7:295, 1991

Triangular Fibrocartilage Tear

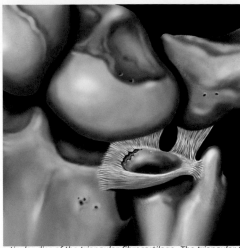

Tear of the articular disc of the triangular fibrocartilage. The triangular fibrocartilage is composed of the dorsal and volar radioulnar ligaments as well as the articular disc.

Key Facts
- Traumatic injuries (Class I)
- Degenerative injuries (Class II)
- Centrum of TFC is thin and is most common site of tear
- Tearing of dorsal or volar margins of the TFC plus centrum (disc) leads to DRUJ instability
- TFC tear = a cause of ulnar-sided wrist pain

Imaging Findings
General Features
- Partial tears and unidirectional flap tears may be undetected on conventional arthrography or arthroscopic injection

MR Findings
- Normal TFC is a biconcave disk of hypointense signal
- Volar margin tears lead to dorsal subluxation
- Dorsal tears associated with volar subluxation
- Radial sided tears: Dorsal to volar orientation
- Volar instability seen on supination in axial plane
- Dorsal instability seen on pronation in axial plane
- Intrasubstance degeneration demonstrated T1 or T2* weighted coronal images
- Partial or complete tears best visualized on FST2-FSE images
- Primary sign of TFC tear is the presence of fluid extension across articular disc or discontinuity
- Partial tears frequently seen with contour irregularities of proximal or distal margins
- Synovitis and chondromalacia of lunate, triquetrum or ulna: Related findings

Triangular Fibrocartilage Tear

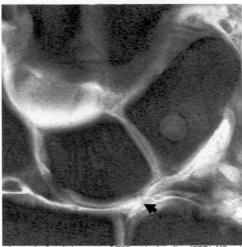

Disruption (arrow) of radial aspect of TFC articular disc (FST1 MR arthrogram).

Differential Diagnosis
Intrasubstance Degeneration
- No hyperintense fluid extension or contour irregularity of TFC

Deformity of TFC without Tear
- Secondary to ulnar minus variance
- Normal hyaline articular cartilage ulnar aspect distal radius
- No fluid signal on FST2-FSE

Tears of Ulnolunate and Ulnotriquetral Ligament

Pathology
General
- General Path Comments
  - Peripheral tears at fovea or radius: Reduced TFC tension with loss of suspensory trampoline effect
  - Attenuated central disc (centrum) site of communications, perforations and tears
  - Perforations related to excessive loading of TFC especially in positive ulnar variance and ulnocarpal abutment syndrome
  - Central perforations (symptomatic) present in 40% by fifth decade, 50% by sixth decade
  - Congenital perforations documented in infants and asymptomatic adults plus degenerative wrists
  - Histological mucinous or myxoid degeneration in degenerative tears
  - Traumatic tears may include injuries to ECU tendon sheath and LT ligament

Clinical Issues
Presentation
- TFC tears associated with positive ulnar variance
- Higher incidence of ulnar-sided tears in younger patients
- Asymptomatic tears increase after age 35

Triangular Fibrocartilage Tear

- Central perforations associated with TFC degeneration and ulnocarpal abutment

Treatment & Prognosis
- Relieve overloading of distal ulna
- Debride/repair tear
- Resection and debridement of flap tear
- Augmentation if repair not possible
- Reconstruction may have better long term results than resection
- Triquetral impingement of ulnar styloid: Treat with a limited ulnar styloidectomy

Selected References
1.   Sugimoto H et al: Triangular fibrocartilage in asymptomatic subjects: Investigations of abnormal signal intensity. Radiology. 191:193, 1994
2.   Katig HS et al: Triangular fibrocartilage and intercarpal ligaments of the wrist: MR imaging. Cadaveric study with gross pathologic and histologic correlation. Radiology. 181:40, 1991
3.   Palmer Ak: Triangular fibrocartilage complex lesions: A classification. J. Hand Surg [Am]. 14:594, 1989

Intraarticular Radius Fractures

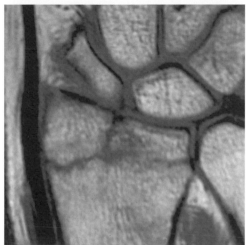

Intraarticular distal radius fracture with fracture segments both perpendicular and parallel to the long axial distal radius (T1-weighted coronal image).

Key Facts
- Frykman classification into intraarticular or extraarticular and involvement of distal radioulnar joint (DRUJ)
- Melone's classification of articular fractures based on the degree and direction of displacement of articular fragments
- Melone's classification indicates when open reduction is required for anatomic reduction
- Linear fracture line extends to distal radius best seen on coronal MR images

Imaging Findings
MR Findings
- Fracture line(s) to distal radius: Hypointense on T1 and hyperintense on FST2-FSE or STIR images
- Associated subchondral edema diffuse hyperintensity on FST2-FSE images
- Synovitis and subcutaneous edema: Associated with fracture
- Fracture diastasis directly measured on coronal, axial or sagittal images
- Scaphoid and lunate fossa evaluated on coronal images
- T2* images may be helpful in identifying fragments if subchondral edema is severe and obscures fracture detail
- Chondral disruption, carpal fractures, ligamentous injuries: Frequent associated findings

Differential Diagnosis
Contusion
No Discrete Fracture Line (no division into segments)
Colles' Fracture
Fracture Line (within 2-3 cm of articular surface distal radius)

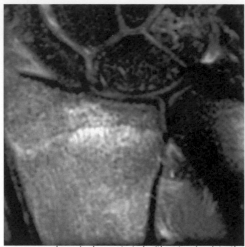

Hyperintense marrow edema is demonstrated with extension into the metaphysis and distal diaphysis (FST2-FSE coronal MR image).

Die Punch Fractures
- Part of spectrum of intraarticular fractures with lunate impaction on the distal radius

Pathology
General
- Etiology-Pathogenesis
  - Fall with impaction
Staging or Grading Criteria
- Melone classification (medial complex at level of lunate fossa)
- Type 1 fracture: Medial complex +/- displaced with stable reduction and congruity
- Type 2 fracture: Comminution is unstable with anterior or posteriorly displaced medial complex
- Type 3 fracture: Medial complex is displaced plus spike fragment
- Type 4 fracture: Separation or rotation of dorsal and palmar medial fragments plus disruption distal radial articular surface

Clinical Issues
Presentation
- Barton fracture: From a fall on an outstretched hand
- Intraarticular unstable fracture dorsal lip distal radius plus carpus follows dorsal fragment
- Reverse Barton's fracture: Intraarticular fracture of the volar lip of the distal radius
- Chauffeur or Hutchinson's fracture: Dorsiflexion and abduction of the hand
- Involves radial styloid
- Incongruity of distal radius greater than 2 mm displacement leads to arthrosis

Intraarticular Radius Fractures

<u>Treatment & Prognosis</u>
- Arthroscopic percutaneous pinning and reduction
- Augmentation from buttressing bone grafts from extraarticular approach

Selected References
1. Melone C Jr. Open treatment for displaced articular fractures of the distal radius. Cln Orthop 1986:202:103

Scaphoid Fracture

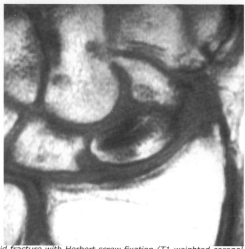

Scaphoid fracture with Herbert screw fixation (T1-weighted coronal image).

Key Facts
- Most common fracture of the carpus
- Associated dorsiflexion loading and radial deviation mechanism
- 70% involved in the middle one-third (scaphoid waist)
- Waist fractures are at risk for delayed union and AVN
- Pain over anatomical snuffbox

Imaging Findings
MR Findings
- Fracture line hypointense on T1-weighted images/acute fracture is hyperintense on T2-weighted images
- Sagittal images show scaphoid flexion (humpback deformity)
- Fracture extension to ulnar or radial cortex differentiates acute from chronic fractures
- Evaluate integrity of scapholunate ligament and volar capsule (RSC and RLT) ligaments
- FST2-FSE or STIR images sensitive to proximal pole edema
Scintigraphy Findings
- Bone scintigraphy may be negative first 48 hours while MR is positive

Differential Diagnosis
Contusion without Fracture Line
Sclerosis Associated with Arthritis
- SLAC or triscaphe

Pathology
General
- Etiology-Pathogenesis
  - Fall on dorsiflexed and outstretched hand
- General Path Comments

Scaphoid Fracture

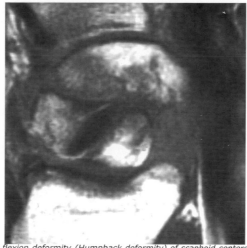

Associated flexion deformity (Humpback deformity) of scaphoid centered at site of waist fracture (T1-weighted sagittal image).

- ○ Transverse fractures (perpendicular to the long axis of the scaphoid) most common and more stable (although all complete fractures are potentially unstable)
- ○ Vertical fractures usually unstable
- ○ Fracture gap 1 mm or less = stable
- ○ Tubercle fractures have good diagnosis
- ○ Blood supply of scaphoid is through distal pole from radial artery branches
- ○ 20% of fractures involve proximal pole
- ○ 10% of fractures involve distal pole
- ○ Proximal pole AVN and delayed healing associated with waist fractures

Clinical Issues
Presentation
- • Pain over anatomical snuffbox
- • Associated dorsiflexion loading and radial deviation mechanism

Treatment & Prognosis
- • Closed or titanium screw
- • Unstable fractures have a non-union rate of 50%
- • Complications: Scaphoid flexion, carpal instability (DISI), arthritis, carpal tunnel syndrome and RSD

Selected References
1. Fernandez DL et al: Non-union of the scaphoid. J Bone Joint Surg [Am]. 77A:883, 1995
2. Duppe H et al: Long-term results of fracture of the scaphoid. J Bone Joint Surg [Am]. 76A:Z4, 1994
3. Smith DK et al. Dorsal lunate tilt (DISI configuration): Sign of scaphoid fracture displacement. Radiology. 176:497, 1990

AVN Scaphoid

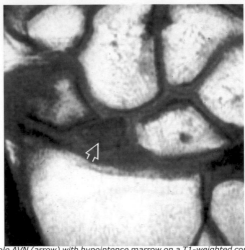

Proximal pole AVN (arrow) with hypointense marrow on a T1-weighted coronal image.

Key Facts
- Secondary to proximal pole or waist fractures
- Proximal pole sclerosis associated with osteopenia and edema
- Necrotic bone hypointense on T1 and hyperintense on FST2-FSE or STIR images in acute and subacute stages

Imaging Findings
MR Findings
- As sensitive as scintigraphy and more specific
- Hypointense signal in the proximal pole on T1 and T2-weighted images is most common MR appearance
- Diffuse necrosis shows marrow signal changes not limited to proximal pole
- Reactive marrow edema of distal pole may not represent necrosis
- IV gadolinium enhances hyperemic tissue
- Lack of proximal pole contrast enhancement related to a lack of vascular perfusion
- Nonunion seen with persistent hyperintensity at fracture site and lack of cortical continuity
- Fluid or fibrous tissue may be present at nonunion site
- Fracture line may remain hypointense although adjacent marrow is hyperintense
- Requires both T1 and FST2-FSE or STIR images to identify edema, fracture line and AVN focus

Imaging Recommendations
- Repeat MRI in 4-6 weeks, may identify persistent proximal pole changes seen in AVN
- Clinical union versus pseudoarthrosis may require CT examination using less than 1 mm sections

AVN Scaphoid

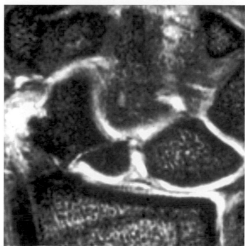

Corresponding T2* coronal image showing the complication of SLAC arthritis with narrowing of the radioscaphoid articulation at the level of the distal pole.

Differential Diagnosis

Preiser's Disease
- AVN of the scaphoid in the absence of a fracture line

Fracture Healing
- With edema hyperintense on T2-weighted images

Pathology

General
- Etiology-Pathogenesis
  - Post traumatic event compromises dominant blood supply of the scaphoid
- General Path Comments
  - Acute fracture may be associated with signal intensity changes in proximal and distal poles which may or may not progress to proximal pole AVN

Clinical Issues

Presentation
- Complication of SLAC arthritis
- Sprain and laxity of RSC (radioscaphocapitate) ligament

Treatment & Prognosis
- Vascularized pedicle graft for scaphoid nonunion with a nonviable proximal fragment

Selected References
1. Fernandez DL et al: Non-union of the scaphoid. J Bone Joint [Am]. 77A:883, 1995
2. Golimbu CN et al: Avascular necrosis of carpal bones. MRI Clin North Am. 3:28, 1995
3. Duppe H et al: Long-term results of fracture of the scaphoid. J Bone Joint Surg [Am]. 76A:249, 1994

Kienböck's Disease

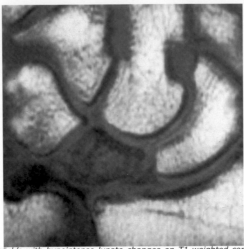

Early Kienböck's with hypointense lunate changes on T1-weighted coronal image. Lunate height is maintained.

Key Facts
- AVN lunate
- Peak age 20 to 40 years with 2:1 male-to-female ratio
- Related to trauma and ulnar negative variance

Imaging Findings
General Features
- Stage I
  - Conventional radiographs normal
  - Bone scintigraphy sensitive and nonspecific
  - Focal or diffuse hypointensity on T1-weighted images
  - STIR or FST2FSE sequences sensitive to hyperemia: vascular dilation
  - Radiocarpal joint effusions and synovitis: Hyperintense on T2-weighted images
  - Hyperemic bone hyperintense on gadolinium-enhanced images
- Stage II
  - Sclerosis on conventional radiograph
  - Hypointense on T1, viable marrow hyperintense on FST2FSE and STIR
  - Decreased height radial aspect lunate stage II disease
- Stage III
  - Distal to proximal collapse in the coronal plane and elongation in the sagittal plane
  - Reciprocal proximal migration of capitate
  - Stage IIIA: Intact scapholunate ligament
  - Stage IIIB: Scapholunate dissociation
  - Scaphoid rotation: Tilts along axis of lunate on coronal images and is equivalent to "ring" sign on conventional radiographs

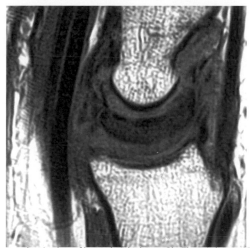

A separate case showing loss of lunate height (stage 3). There is lunate AP elongation in the sagittal plane.

- Stage IV
  - Degenerative arthrosis of the lunate and carpus
  - Lunate hypointense on all pulse sequences
  - Lunate collapse in all three orthogonal planes

Differential Diagnosis
Clinical Differential
- Dorsal ganglion, RA, degenerative arthritis, synovitis, and fracture
Imaging Differential
- Ulnar impaction syndrome
Sclerosis (eccentric and ulnar in location)

Pathology
General
- Etiology-Pathogenesis
  - Fractures and trauma may disrupt intraosseous blood supply and lead to AVN
  - Correlation with negative ulnar variance with lunate subjected to increased mechanical loading

Clinical Issues
Presentation
- Age 20–40 years, unilateral presentation more common
- Dorsal tenderness about lunate
- Stiffness secondary to synovitis
- Carpal tunnel syndrome
- Weakness and decreased grip strength
Treatment & Prognosis
- Early stages: Unload and revascularize the lunate
- Later stages treated with arthrodesis and salvage procedures

Kienböck's Disease

Selected References
1. Watanabe K et al: Imaeda T. Arthroscopic assessment of Kienböck's disease. Arthroscopy. 2:257, 1995
2. Desser TS et al: Scaphoid fractures and Kienböck's disease of the lunate: MR imaging with histopathologic correlation. Magn Reson Imaging. 8:357, 1990
3. Beckenbaugh R et al: Kienböck's disease: the natural history of Kienböck's disease and consideration of lunate fractures. Clin Orthop. 149:98, 1980

Carpal Tunnel Syndrome

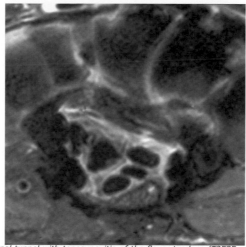

Carpal tunnel with tenosynovitis of the flexor tendons (T2FSE axial).

Key Facts
- Compromise of motor and/or sensory function of median nerve at the level of the carpal tunnel
- Secondary to trauma (including repetitive wrist activities), hemorrhage, infection, and infiltrative disease
- Pain and numbness: Thumb, index, middle fingers and radial ½ of the ring finger most commonly affected

Imaging Findings
MR Findings
- Swelling or segmental enlargement of median nerve at level of pisiform
- Flattening of median nerve at level of hamate
- Palmar bowing of flexor retinaculum at level of hamate
- Hyperintensity of median nerve on T2-weighted images
- Fibrosis of median nerve is hypointense on T1 and T2-weighed images
- Incomplete release of flexor retinaculum associated with residual nerve hyperintensity
- Pseudoneuroma-swelling of median nerve proximal to carpal tunnel

Differential Diagnosis
Colles' Fracture
- Associated with decreased volume of carpal tunnel
Inflammatory Processes
- Rheumatoid arthritis, gout, pseudogout, and amyloid-type inflammatory processes with decreased carpal tunnel volume
Median Nerve Tumors
- Neurilemomas, fibromas, and hamartomas
Tumors Extrinsic To Median Nerve
- Ganglia, lipomas, and hemangiomas (space occupying)
Endocrine Disorders
- Diabetes mellitus, hypothyroidism, pregnancy, and lupus

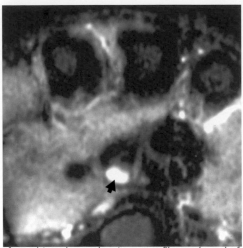

Symptoms of carpal tunnel secondary to a neurofibroma (arrow) of the median nerve. (hyperintense on STIR axial image).

Pathology
General
- Etiology-Pathogenesis
  - Secondary to trauma (including repetitive wrist activities), hemorrhage, infection, and infiltrative disease
  - Increased pressure in carpal tunnel
  - Compression or swelling of median nerve in its synovial sheath
- Nerve ischemia: Progressive stages of venous congestion, nerve edema, venous and arterial compromise

Clinical Issues
Presentation
- Between 30 and 60 years of age
- Female to male ratio 325:1
- 50% of cases bilateral
- Pain and numbness: Thumb, index, middle fingers and radial ½ of the ring finger most commonly affected
- Increased nocturnal pain and/or burning plus pain and numbness
- Sensory findings: Minimal, hypesthesia to complete anesthesia
- Muscle atrophy and loss of function late findings
- Abductor pollicis brevis muscle early involvement
- Positive Tinel's sign indicates nerve entrapment (tingling) in digits supplied by median nerve

Treatment & Prognosis
- Conservative: Initial
- Surgical decompression for progressive sensory loss and muscle atrophy plus weakness

Carpal Tunnel Syndrome

Selected References

1.   Sugimoto H et al: Carpal tunnel syndrome: Evaluation of median nerve circulation with dynamic contrast-enhanced MR imaging. Radiology. 190:459, 1994
2.   Mesgarzadah M et al: Carpal tunnel: MR imaging. Part 1. Normal anatomy. Radiology. 171:743, 1989
3.   Mesgarzadah M et al: Carpal tunnel: MR imaging. Part II. Carpal tunnel syndrome. Radiology. 171:749, 1989

Ulnar Collateral Ligament Tear

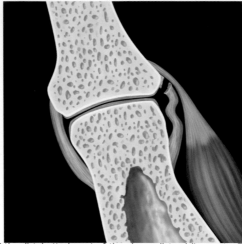

Rupture of the distal attachment of the ulnar collateral ligament. The adductor aponeurosis is superficial to the UCL.

Key Facts
- Gamekeeper's thumb: Disruption of the ulnar collateral ligament (usually involving the distal attachment to the proximal phalanx)
- Associated with a proximal phalanx base fracture
- Instability with abduction stress
- Stener lesion: Ulnar collateral ligament (UCL) relocates superficial to adductor pollicis aponeurosis

Imaging Findings
MR Findings
- Edema, thickening, disruption, displacement or entrapment of ulnar collateral ligament
- Torn ulnar collateral ligament remains deep to overlying adductor aponeurosis
- FST2FSE or STIR useful in identifying edema and osseous contusion
- T2* useful in showing torn ligament and any avulsed osseous fragment
- Primary MR diagnosis on coronal images through the metacarpophalangeal joint with secondary diagnosis performed in axial plane
- Retracted ligament is thickened proximally with medial bowing of adductor aponeurosis

Differential Diagnosis
Ulnar Collateral Ligament Sprain
- There is continuity of ligament to bone
- Partial tear also at distal ligament attachment

Pathology
General
- Etiology-Pathogenesis
  - Forceful abduction of thumb

Ulnar Collateral Ligament Tear

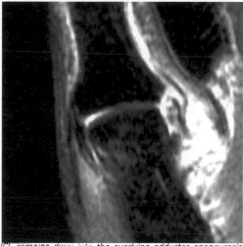

Retracted UCL remains deep into the overlying adductor aponeurosis. No Stener lesion is present (STIR coronal image).

Clinical Issues

Presentation

- Commonly seen in football, hockey, wrestling and basketball injuries
- Also skier's thumb abduction injury with ski poles
- Metacarpophalangeal joint instability with at least 20 degrees greater laxity vs contralateral thumb

Treatment & Prognosis

- The Stener lesion requires surgical treatment

Selected References
1. Noszian IM et al: Ulnar collateral ligament: differentiation of displaced and nondisplaced tears with US. Radiology. 194:61, 1995
2. Hinkle DHet al: Ulnar collateral ligament of the thumb: MR findings in cadavers, volunteers and patients with ligamentous injury (gamekeeper's thumb). AJR. 163:1431, 1994
3. Spaeth HJ et al: Gamekeeper thumb: Differentiation of nondisplaced and displaced tears of the ulnar collateral ligament with MR imaging. Radiology. 188:553, 1993

HIP

AVN Femoral Head

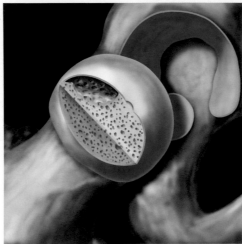

AVN of the femoral head involving the superior weightbearing portion (anterolateral portion) of the femoral head.

Key Facts
- Related to trauma: Displaced femoral neck fracture and less commonly status post fracture or dislocation of the hip
- Disrupted vascular supply at time of injury
- Non-traumatic AVN occurs in younger population and is bilateral
- MR sensitive to changes of marrow fat signal intensity

Imaging Findings
Plain Film Findings
- Subchondral collapse (advanced) sign seen as a subarticular radiolucent crescent in the anterosuperior femoral head
- Involvement of femoral head greater than involvement of joint space changes (narrowing) or acetabular findings
- Femoral head sclerosis
Scintigraphy Findings
- Early detection relative to conventional radiographs (less sensitive relative to MR)
- Technetium labeled phosphate analogues and sulfur colloid
CT Findings
- Sclerotic pattern on axial CT images
- More accurate than conventional radiographs for staging
- Less sensitive relative to MR
MR Findings
- More sensitive than CT or bone scintigraphy
- Articular cartilage intact at presentation
- Wedge-shaped subchondral bone infarct
- Sagittal images used to assess femoral head morphology for cortical flattening (routine imaging with coronal and axial images)
- Double line sign in 80% (hyperintense inner border parallel to hypointense periphery on T2-weighted images)

AVN Femoral Head

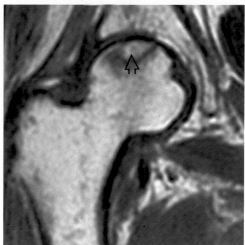

Left femoral head AVN (arrow) with central fat marrow signal preserved (T1-weighted coronal image).

- Staging Ficat and Arlet
  - Stage 1: Trabeculae normal to porotic +/- double line sign
  - Stage 2: Sclerosis of trabeculae
  - Stage 3: Loss of spherical shape of femoral head
  - Stage 4: Collapse of femoral head, articular cartilage destruction and joint space narrowing
- Mitchell MR classifications: Qualitative assessment of alterations in the central region of MR signal intensity in osteonecrotic focus
- Decreased enhancement with gadolinium in early AVN
- Double line sign
- Femoral head plus neck edema
- Fibrous replacement hypointense on T1 and T2

Differential Diagnosis
Capital Fracture and/or Contusion
- No double line sign

Bone Marrow Edema without Reactive Interface

Pathology
General
- General Path Comments
  - Ineffective healing response with bone reabsorption of ischemic focus
  - Unsupported articular cartilage secondary to subchondral fracture leads to joint destruction
  - Central region of hyperintensity equals necrosis of bone and marrow prior to capillary mesenchymal ingrowth
  - Hypointense peripheral band equals sclerotic margin of reactive tissue at necrotic and viable bone interface
  - Double line sign: Inflammatory response with granulation tissue inside reactive bone interface

- Etiology-Pathogenesis
  o Related to trauma: Displaced femoral neck fracture and less commonly status post fracture or dislocation of the hip
  o Disrupted vascular supply at time of injury

Clinical Issues

Presentation

- Often associated with asymptomatic contralateral involvement (increased risk of contralateral AVN)
- Hip or groin pain +/- referred thigh or knee pain
- Decreased hip rotation and range of motion (this may be increased by the presence of a joint effusion)

Treatment & Prognosis

- Core decompression +/- bone grafts, osteotomy and electrical stimulation for treatment
- Decrease in elevated intraosseous pressure with core decompression to permit neovascularization
- Core decompression used for grade I and II: Best results with less than 25% involvement of weightbearing surface of the femoral head

Selected References
1. Beltran J et al: Femoral head avascular necrosis: MR imaging with clinical-pathologic and radionuclide correlation. Radiology. 166:215, 1988
2. Mitchell DG et al: Femoral head avascular necrosis: Correlation of MR imaging, radiographic staging, radionuclide imaging and clinical findings. Radiology. 162:709, 1987
3. Totty WG et al: Magnetic resonance imaging of the normal and ischemic femoral head. AJR AM J Roentgenol. 143:1273-80, 1984

Legg-Calvé-Perthes

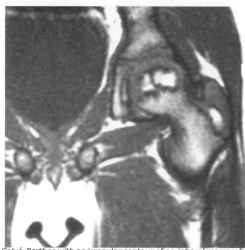

Early Legg-Calvé-Perthes with an irregular contour of peripheral marrow fat-containing epiphyseal ossification center (T1-weighted coronal image).

Key Facts
- Infarction of bony epiphysis of femoral head
- Age range 4-8 years (most susceptible for femoral head vascular supply)
- M:F = 5:1
- Asymmetric distribution with 10% bilateral
- Limp with groin, thigh or knee pain (referred)
- Hypointensity capital epiphysis on coronal MR images

Imaging Findings
Plain Film Findings
- Effusion, fragmentation and flattening of sclerotic capital epiphysis and metaphyseal irregularity (rarefaction of lateral and medial metaphysis and cystic changes)
- Joint space (inferomedial) widening with intact articular subchondral plate
- Catterall classification (Group I-IV) estimates amount of femoral head involvement
Scintigraphy Findings
- Early decrease secondary to interruption of blood supply
- Increased uptake seen late with secondary revascularization and repair and degenerative arthritis
MR Findings
- Hypointense epiphyseal marrow center on T1 and T2-weighted images
- Associated findings: Intraarticular effusion, hypoplastic laterally displaced ossification nucleus
- Hypointense irregularity along periphery of ossific nucleus or linear hypointense traversing femoral ossification center in early stages (stage I)
- Revascularization of necrotic epiphysis post treatment seen with replacement of hypointense focus with marrow fat

Legg-Calvé-Perthes

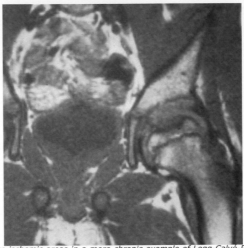

Hypointense ischemic areas in a more chronic example of Legg-Calvé-Perthes (T1-weighted coronal image).

- Coxa plana and coxa magna: Late remodeling
- FST2-FSE images to assess articular cartilage thickness and chondral irregularities
- Physeal cartilage +/- hyperintensity on T2-weighted images: Early stage disease
- Loss of femoral head containment in acetabulum: Hypertrophied synovium in iliopsoas recess and thickening of epiphyseal cartilage
- Sagittal images supplement coronal plane in displaying acetabular and femoral head cartilage

Differential Diagnosis
Infection
- Greater soft-tissue reaction and/or inhomogeneous effusion
Erosion of Subchondral Plate in Capital Epiphysis
Irritable Hip
- No marrow necrosis

Pathology
General
- Etiology-Pathogenesis
  o Insufficiency of capital epiphysis blood supply with physis acting as a barrier
  o Overgrowth articular cartilage medially and laterally
  o Trabecular fracture with decreased epiphyseal height: Infarction
  o Disease progressive

Clinical Issues
Presentation
- Risk factors
- Flexion and abduction contracture
- Lateral overgrowth of epiphysis cartilage and loss of abduction

Legg-Calvé-Perthes

Treatment & Prognosis
- 50% improved with no treatment
- Younger age of presentation equals better prognosis (greater than 8 years old equals poor prognosis)
- Girls: More severe form
- Epiphyseal signs (calcification lateral to epiphysis + lytic area laterally) and metaphyseal (horizontal inclination of growth plate) signs associated with poor prognosis
- Bracing or femoral osteotomy
- 86% develop osteoarthritis
- Increased epiphyseal extrusion at greater than 20% = poor prognosis
- Greater than 50% femoral head involvement = poor prognosis

Selected References
1. Rush BH et al: Legg-Calvé-Perthes disease: Detection of cartilaginous and synovial changes with MR imaging. Radiology. 167:473, 1988
2. Haston EJ Jr et al: Magnetic resonance imaging and scintigraphy in Legg-Perthes' disease: Diagnosis, treatment and prognosis. Radiology. 165:35, 1987
3. Catterall A et al: A review of the morphology of Perthes disease. J Bone Joint Surg [Br]. 64:269, 1982

Developmental Dysplasia of Hip

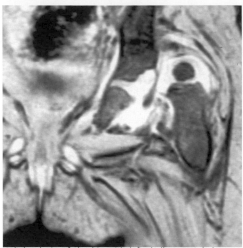

Developmental dysplasia of the hip with left shallow acetabulum and dislocated capital epiphysis and deformed everted labrum (T2* coronal image).

Key Facts
- Acetabular dysplasia and superolateral migration of the femoral head
- Hypoplasia capital epiphysis
- Labral irregularities plus MR findings of labral coverage of capital epiphysis
- Left hip involvement: 40-60%
- Bilateral involvement: 20%
- Infants at risk: Positive family history, breech, torticollis, scoliosis, metatarsus adductus

Imaging Findings
Plain Film Findings
- False negative diagnosis less than six weeks
- Femoral capital epiphysis located in inner lower quadrant based on Hilgenreiner's line through triradiate cartilage and Perkins' line (perpendicular to Hilgenreiner's) through lateral acetabular rim
- Lateral subluxation of capital epiphysis with measurement of 2 mm or greater from teardrop to metaphysis
- Superior subluxation with measurement of delta of 2 mm or greater from Hilgenreiner's line to metaphysis
- Disruption of Shenton's curved line: Formed by inferior aspect superior pubic ramus
- Center edge angle less than 25 degrees: Associated with instability
- Secondary signs
  - Acetabular dysplasia
  - Excessive femoral head anteversion
  - Delayed ossification of capital epiphysis
Ultrasound Findings
- Up to 8 to 10 months: Application of ultrasound
- Visualized iliac bone, acetabulum, labrum and femoral capital epiphysis

Developmental Dysplasia of Hip

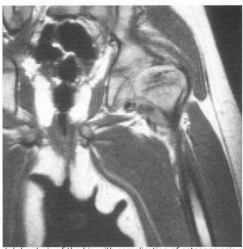

Developmental dysplasia of the hip with complication of osteonecrosis of the capital epiphysis (T1-weighted coronal image).

- Evaluate subluxation, dislocation, pulvinar, inverted labrum, hypoplastic ossific nucleus, acetabular dysplasia and ossification and alpha angle (between lateral edge of ilium and bony acetabular margin: abnormal angle less than 50 degrees at birth and 50-59 degrees at three months of age)

CT Findings
- Use coronal and axial CT images or reformations
- Sector angle for acetabular coverage (capital epiphysis to acetabular rim relative to the horizontal axis)

MR Findings
- Epiphyseal articular cartilage intermediate signal intensity on T1-weighted images and hyperintense on T2*-weighted images (gradient echo technique)
- Coronal and axial images identify position of capital epiphysis
- Useful when ossific nucleus not visible on conventional radiographs or CT
- Ischemic necrosis use T1- and T2-weighted images
- Effusions hyperintense on T2-weighted images
- Failure to reduce
  - o Hourglass acetabulum, inverted labrum
  - o Interposed iliopsoas tendon (seen on coronal, axial and sagittal images)
  - o Direct visualization of pulvinar fibrofatty tissue and hypertrophy of ligamentum teres
- Superolateral dislocation use coronal plane images
- AP relationship and dysplasia of acetabulum use axial plane images
- Acetabular labral coverage lateral to dysplastic acetabulum-use coronal images
- Long term follow-up
- Subsequent evaluation for development of osteoarthritis

Developmental Dysplasia of Hip

- Acetabular index calculation from coronal MR (Hilgenreiner's line through triradiate cartilage and tangent through acetabular roof greater than 30 degrees)

Differential Diagnosis
Proximal Focal Femoral Deficiency
- Shortening the proximal segment of the femur

Coxa Vara
- Neck to shaft angle less than 120 degrees

Slipped Capital Femoral Epiphysis
- Capital epiphysis maintains acetabular coverage

Pathology
General
- Etiology-Pathogenesis
  - Laxity of joint capsule ligament
  - Mechanical versus physiologic (elevated maternal estrogen levels)
  - Hourglass joint capsule: Compression between limbus and ligamentum teres
  - Type 1: Positional instability
  - Type 2: Subluxation
  - Type 3: Dislocation

Clinical Issues
Presentation
- Incidence: 0.15% of neonates
- Ortolani's test: Dislocated capital epiphysis (hip abduction at 90 degrees flexion plus anterior pressure relocates femoral head)
- Barlow's test: Dislocatable hip (unstable femoral head dislocated by posterior pressure)

Treatment & Prognosis
- Closed reduction
- Abductor tenotomy and release of iliopsoas
- Open reduction
- Varus osteotomy (derotational)
- Reconstructive osteotomy
  - Pemberton acetabuloplasty (from anterior inferior iliac spine to triradiate cartilage)
  - Salter opening wedge (from anterior inferior iliac spine across sacrosciatic notch)
  - Triple innominate osteotomy (skeletally mature patient with osteotomy across iliac neck, pubis and ischium)
  - Chiari-medialization of femoral head as a salvage procedure (osteotomy across superior acetabulum)

Selected References
1. Eggli KO et al: Low-Dose CT of developmental dysplasia of the hip after reduction: Diagnostic accuracy and dosimetry. AJR. 163:1441, 1994
2. Atar D et al: 2-D and 3-D computed tomography and magnetic resonance imaging in developmental dysplasia of the hip. Orthopedic Review. 1189, 1992
3. Johnson ND et al: Complex infantile and congenital hip dislocation: Assessment with MR imaging. Radiology. 168:151, 1988

Muscle Strain

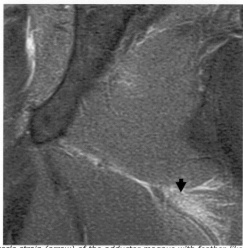

Grade I muscle strain (arrow) of the adductor magnus with feather-like distribution of interstitial muscle edema (FST2-FSE coronal image).

Key Facts
- Indirect injury secondary to excessive stretch
- Overuse microtrauma
- Corresponding pain occurs during or immediately following muscle contraction
- Muscle and myotendinitis tears
- Strains (grading I, II, and III)

Imaging Findings
MR Findings
- Grade I
  - Edema and/or hemorrhage with preservation of muscle morphology
  - Interstitial hyperintensity with feathery distribution hyperintense on T2, fat suppressed T2FSE and STIR images
  - Subcutaneous tissue edema as well as intermuscular fluid
- Grade II
  - Strain or tear, hemorrhage with tearing of up to 50% of muscle fibers
  - Interstitial hyperintensity with focal hyperintensity of hemorrhage in muscle belly +/- the presence of intramuscular fluid
  - Focal defect at tear site with partial retraction of muscle fibers
  - Subacute hemorrhage hyperintense on T1-weighted images
  - Associated myotendinous and tendinous injuries (increased signal intensity with interruption and/or widening of the muscle-tendon-unit or tendon)
- Grade III
  - Complete tearing +/- muscle retraction
  - Fluid filled gap identified as hyperintense on fat suppressed T2FSE and STIR sequences
  - Interstitial muscle changes also present

Muscle Strain

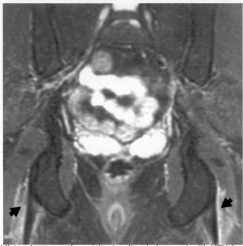

Associated bilateral common hamstring tendinosis (arrows) with MTU (muscle tendon unit) involvement (FST2-FSE coronal image).

    ○   Identify course of retracted muscle fibers (muscle atrophy and/or hypertrophy secondary to retraction)

Differential Diagnosis
- Grade I and DOMS overlap in MR signal intensity changes

DOMS (Delayed Onset Muscle Soreness)
- Nonacute injury
- Painful symptoms increased first 24 hours after exertion and peak 24 to 72 hours then subside
- Denervation demonstrates diffuse muscle group involvement with hyperintense signal best visualized on either STIR or fat suppressed fast spin echo images
- Interstitial hemorrhage and hematoma
- Associated with muscle injury +/- increased in muscle size
- Grade I and DOMS overlap in MR signal intensity changes

Muscle Contusion
- Compressive or concussive direct trauma
- Direct trauma identify associated hematoma in blunt injuries and lacerations from penetrating injuries
- Fluid collections: May cause swelling and weakness
- Muscle contracture and rhabdomyolysis
- Associated with metabolic disorders (coexistence of muscle edema, atrophy and fatty infiltration relates to a myopathic or neurogenic disorder)

Infection
- Fluid collection hyperintense or intermediate on fat suppressed T2FSE or STIR images which may be focal or track superficially

Pathology
General
- Etiology-Pathogenesis
  - ○   Indirect injury secondary to excessive stretch

Muscle Strain

- o Overuse microtrauma
- o Muscle and myotendinitis tears
- o Eccentric loading
- o Strains in the area of highest proportion of fast-twitch type II muscle fibers (e.g. rectus femoris, biceps femoris and medial head gastrocnemius)
- o Muscle-tendon-unit (MTU) equals weakest biomechanical link

Clinical Issues

Presentation

- Weakness absent in primary strain: No myofascial disruption (inflammatory cell infiltrate, edema and swelling)
- Secondary strain: Weakness plus separation of muscle from tendon or fascia
- Third-degree strain: Complete myofascial separation and loss of function
- Rectus femoris strain
- Sprinting or kicking sports
- Mid muscle belly strain +/- chronic pseudocyst in deep intramuscular tendon
- Hamstring muscle strain +/- degeneration and/or partial tear of the conjoined tendon attachment to the posterolateral aspect of ischial tuberosity
- Proximal muscle hamstring injury is most frequent site of involvement
- Incomplete to complete extension of injury
- Fibrosis, fatty replacement, muscle ossification, compartment syndrome

Treatment & Prognosis

- Treatment of small fascial or tendinous tears is conservative
- Rupture of muscle: Possible surgical management
- Fibrosis and retraction of muscle impairment of functional result

Selected References
1. Brandser EA et al: Hamstring injuries: Radiographic, conventional tomographic CT and MR imaging characteristics. Radiology. 197:257, 1995
2. Hasselman CT et al: An explanation for various rectus femoris strain injuries using previously undescribed muscle architecture. AM J Sports Med. 123:493, 1995
3. Doons GC et al: MR imaging of intramuscular hemorrhage. J Comput Assist Tomogr 9:908, 1985

Femoral Neck Fracture

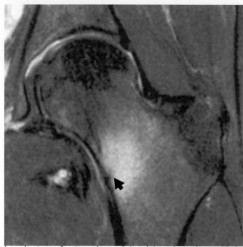

Left femoral neck stress fracture (arrow) involving the calcar with hyperintensity (FST2-FSE).

Key Facts
- Intracapsular femoral neck fractures
  - Subcapital (common) transcervical (uncommon) or basocervical (uncommon)
- Post-traumatic osteonecrosis up to 30%: More common in proximal femoral neck fractures
- Femoral neck stress fractures
  - Overuse with repeated stress to normal bone
  - Insufficiency fractures in osteoporosis

Imaging Findings
Plain Film Findings
- Subcapital fracture
  - Disruption of trabecular pattern, sclerosis secondary to impaction
  - Cortex abnormality at junction of head and neck
  - Frank cortex disruption +/- angulation
- Stress fracture
  - Normal findings on conventional radiographs
  - Sclerosis
  - Blickenstaff and Morris classification
    - Type I: Endosteal or periosteal callus without fracture line
    - Type II: Fracture line
    - Type III: Displaced
MR Findings
- Nondisplaced femoral neck fractures with negative conventional radiographs
- Morphology of fracture segment defined (bone scans nonspecific)
- Microtrabecular stress fracture with intact medial and lateral cortices
- FST2-FSE or STIR images (T1-weighted images also important in defining fat signal intensity versus hypointense fracture line)
- Fracture line may be hypointense on both T1- and T2-weighted images

Femoral Neck Fracture

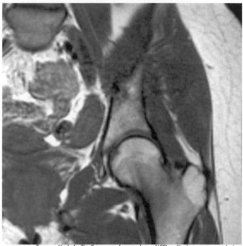

Hypointense area of medial left femoral neck: difficult to appreciate as a stress fracture on corresponding T1-weighted coronal image.

- Adjacent edema and hemorrhage identified with increased signal intensity on fat suppressed T2-FSE and STIR images
- Contrast enhanced MR: Assess femoral head perfusion status post femoral neck fractures with uniform increased signal intensity with intact perfusion
- Differentiate osteoporotic insufficiency fractures versus pathologic fractures (associated marrow replacement)
- Early detection of AVN
- Direct visualization of associated chondral lesions in the acetabulum and femoral head

Differential Diagnosis
Contusion
- Without discrete fracture line

Marrow Replacement
- May be seen with disorder, metastatic disease or primary neoplasia (no discrete fracture line unless complicated by pathologic fracture)

AVN of Femoral Head
- With extended pattern of neck edema without discrete fracture line

Osteoarthritis of the Hip
- With pattern of femoral head and neck edema without discrete fracture line

Transient Osteoporosis of the Hip
- Without identified fracture line

Pathology
General
- Etiology-Pathogenesis
  - Fall with impact on greater trochanter plus lateral rotation of femur
  - Cyclic loading and microfracture with addition of torsional injury
  - Direct diaphysis trauma

Femoral Neck Fracture

- General Path Comments
  - Classification
    - Pauwels' (direction of fracture angle)
    - Garden system (degree of displacement)

Clinical Issues
Presentation
- Intracapsular fracture 2 x more common than trochanteric fracture
- Healing: 6-12 months
- Complications: Delayed union and nonunion, AVN (10-30%)

Treatment & Prognosis
- Stress fracture – conservative treatment
- Knowles pinning
- Endoprosthesis

Selected References
1. May DA et al: MR imaging of occult traumatic fractures and muscular injuries of the hip and pelvis in elderly patients. AJR. 166:1075, 1996
2. Lang P et al: Acute fracture of the femoral neck: Assessment of femoral head. Perfusion with gadopentetate dimeglumine-enhanced MR imaging. AJR. 160:335, 1993
3. Deutsch AL et al: Occult fractures of the proximal femur: MR imaging. Radiology. 170(1): 113, 1989

Labral Tear

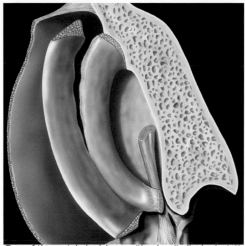

Tear of the acetabular labrum with a longitudinal orientation.

Key Facts

- Surface coil imaging required for small FOVs
- Normal labrum: Triangular in cross section
- Symptoms: Pain, decreased range of motion and clicking
- Increased signal intensity or disruption on FST2-FSE or STIR images
- MR arthrography improves visualization of labral tear

Imaging Findings

<u>MR Findings</u>

- Normal labrum
  - Hypointense
  - Covers hyaline articular cartilage lateral peripheral margin acetabulum
  - Perilabral sulcus around periphery of labrum
  - Thinning of labrum anteroinferiorly
  - Nonvascularized
- Linear hyperintensity in contrast to hypointense labrum on fat-suppressed T2FSE or STIR images
- Associated paralabral cyst: Use FST2-FSE or STIR images (+/- septations or lobulations)
- Surface irregularities associated with base of labrum degeneration
- Czerny classification: Based on MR arthrography (91% sensitive, 71% specific)
  - Stage IA: Hyperintense signal with no communication to articular surface with visualized perilabral sulcus
  - Stage IB: No perilabral sulcus visualized
  - Stage IIA: Contrast extension into articular surface with visualized perilabral sulcus
  - Stage IIB: No perilabral sulcus
  - Stage IIIA: Labral detachment with triangular shape maintained and visualized perilabral sulcus

Labral Tear

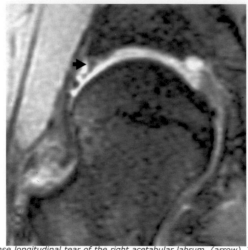

Hyperintense longitudinal tear of the right acetabular labrum. (arrow). T2* coronal image.

- ○ Stage IIIB: Laral detachment and thickened labrum with labral hyperintensity and no perilabral sulcus
- ○ Anterosuperior: Most common location for tears

Differential Diagnosis

Sublabral Foramen

Degenerative Labrum

Normal Acetabular Articular Cartilage

- At interface of medial labrum
- Not hyperintense on T2-weighted images

Normal Fibrovascular Bundles or Irregular Insertion of Labrum

- May mimic degeneration or tear

Pathology

General

- General Path Comments
  - ○ Degenerative changes of the labrum include eosinophilic, mucinous and mucoid changes
  - ○ Cysts (paralabral cysts) occur in a superior anterior or superior posterior location and are hyperintense on T2-weighed images

Clinical Issues

Presentation

- Pain, snapping, clicking and locking
- 28% asymptomatic patient have labral abnormalities
- Labral tears associated with trauma, DDH and osteoarthritis
- Associated early arthritis at the acetabulum may include acetabular roof edema, sclerosis and subchondral cyst development

Treatment & Prognosis

- Debridement
- Modified Bankart

Selected References
1. Leunig M et al: Evaluation of the acetabular labrum by MR arthrography. J Bone Joint Surg Br. 79B: 230-4, 1997
2. Petersilge CA et al: Acetabular labral tears: Evaluation with MR arthrography. Radiology. 200:231-5, 1996
3. Lecouver FE et al: MR imaging of the acetabular labrum: Variations in 200 asymptomatic hips. AJR Am J Roentgenol. 167:1025-8, 1996

Transient Osteoporosis

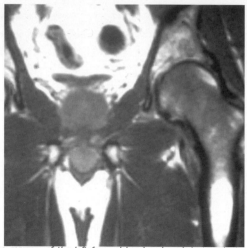

Hypointense marrow of the left femoral head and neck in transient osteoporosis (T1-weighted coronal image).

Key Facts
- Self-limiting and unknown etiology
- Women in third trimester (original description) involving left hip
- Middle-aged males (M>F)
- Progressive hip and groin pain with decreased range of motion and limp in absence of infection or trauma
- Effusion and progressive demineralization of femoral neck and acetabulum
- Involvement of one joint at a time
- Joint space preserved

Imaging Findings
MR Findings
- Prior to conventional radiographic signs are seen
  - Diffuse marrow edema (partial femoral head sparing also seen) of femoral head and neck with hypointensity on T1 and hyperintensity on FST2-FSE and STIR images
  - Hyperintense effusion on T2-weighted images (FST2-FSE)
  - Marrow edema may extend to intertrochanteric line
  - No subchondral sclerosis or fracture in superior femoral head
  - Mild acetabular signal intensity changes similar to findings in the femoral head
  - Resolution of MR abnormalities in 6-10 months

Differential Diagnosis
AVN
- Subchondral fracture is present
- Bone marrow edema syndrome thought to represent initial phase of nontraumatic AVN although high-resolution imaging with MR usually identifies subchondral fractures in true ischemia

Reflex Sympathetic Dystrophy
- Subchondral signal changes

Transient Osteoporosis

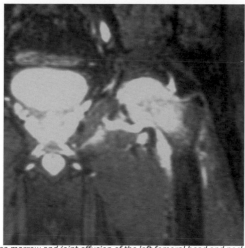

Hyperintense marrow and joint effusion of the left femoral head and neck in transient osteoporosis. Note no subchondral fracture is present (STIR coronal image).

Regional Migratory Osteoporosis
- No demineralization present

Inflammatory Osteoarthritis
- Joint space narrowing and the presence of sclerosis

Septic Arthritis
- May demonstrate inhomogeneity of signal intensity secondary to synovial tissue and debris

Metastases
- Trabecular destruction can be documented on CT bone technique

Pathology
General
- Etiology-Pathogenesis
  - Self-limiting and unknown etiology
  - Effusion and progressive demineralization of femoral neck and acetabulum

Microscopic Features
- Normal marrow (with the presence of edema) and bone without histologic evidence of ischemia
- Elevation of pressure within bone marrow
- Transient bone marrow edema: More comprehensive term (conventional radiographs may be insensitive to early demineralization)

Clinical Issues
Presentation
- More common in men
- Affects right or left side +/- migration from one side to the other
- Pain, restricted motion and limp

Treatment & Prognosis
- Self-limited

Transient Osteoporosis

Selected References

1. Bloem JL: Transient osteoporosis of the hip: MR imaging. Radiology. 167:753-5, 1998
2. Guerra JJ et al: Distinguishing transient osteoporosis from avascular necrosis of the hip. J Bone Joint Surg Am. 77A: 616-24, 1995
3. Hayes CW et al: MR imaging of bone marrow edema pattern: transient osteoporosis, transient bone marrow edema or osteonecrosis. Radiographics. 13:1001-11, 1993

Osteoarthritis (Hip)

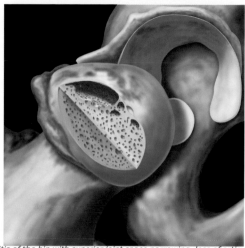

Osteoarthritis of the hip with superior joint space narrowing, loss of articular cartilage and subchondral cystic change.

Key Facts
- Most common form articular cartilage degeneration
- Primary and secondary (old SCFE, dysplasia, Legg-Calvé-Perthes)
- Painful weight bearing and decreased range of motion
- Early findings with MR include acetabular roof sclerosis, subchondral edema and cystic changes prior to positive conventional radiographs
- Loss of joint space
- Osteophytes

Imaging Findings
Plain Film & CT Findings
- Superior or superolateral migration femoral head (80%)
- Medial migration plus protrusio acetabuli (20%)
- Egger's cyst of acetabulum
- Calcar buttressing
- Ring of osteophytes (lateral acetabulum and medial subcapital)
- Sclerosis of femoral head and acetabular roof

MR Findings
- Focal loss of articular cartilage
- Chondral fissures or hyperintensity in acetabular roof articular cartilage especially superolateral with the association of early subchondral sclerosis of the acetabular roof
- Paralabral cysts and lateral acetabular rim cysts
- T1, FST2-FSE with 16 to 18 cm FOV to assess chondral surfaces
- Stress: Thickened trabeculae hypointense on T1 and T2-weighted images
- Small subchondral cysts hyperintense on T2-weighted images (FST2-FSE and STIR) prior to superior joint-space narrowing, lateral acetabular and femoral head osteophytes and medial buttressing
- May be seen in association with AVN

Osteoarthritis (Hip)

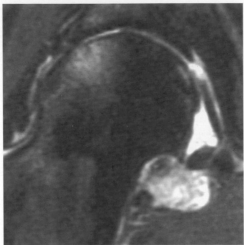

Inflammatory osteoarthritis with superior joint space narrowing, capsular synovitis and subchondral edema of acetabular roof and weightbearing femoral head. Osteophytes of the femoral head-neck junction are present (FST2-FSE coronal image).

- IV or intraarticular contrast: Use to evaluate synovium and assess chondral surfaces
- Associated joint effusions hyperintense on T2-weighted images

Differential Diagnosis
Hernation Pit
- Anterosuperior aspect lateral femoral neck (not part of OA spectrum)
- Secondary to pressure effects of anterior hip capsule
AVN
- Greater involvement of femoral head prior to joint space narrowing
- Articular cartilage thickness initially maintained
Rheumatoid Variants
- Medial migration (less common for osteoarthritis) and erosions plus concentric narrowing
Pseudogout or PVNS
- Large cyst formation
Inflammatory Osteoarthritis
- May mimic infection or AVN

Pathology
General
- Etiology-Pathogenesis
  - Excessive stress on normal tissue or abnormal response to normal forces
  - Inflammation contributes to cartilage degeneration
- Staging or Grading Criteria
  - Grade I: Chondral inhomogeneity
  - Grade II: Inhomogeneity plus discontinuity of chondral surface, hypointensity of femoral head and neck and loss of trabecular detail on T1

- o Grade III: Grade II changes plus irregular cortical morphology of femoral head and acetabulum plus cystic changes of the femoral head plus indistinct zone between femoral head and acetabulum
- o Grade IV: The addition of femoral head deformity

Clinical Issues
Presentation
- Incidence of OA increases with age
- Early acetabular chondral and subchondral changes may be seen in younger patients ages 30-50 prior to femoral head findings: These early OA changes may be secondary to trauma

Treatment & Prognosis
- Intraarticular steroids
- Anti-inflammatory nonsteroidal
- Total joint arthroplasty

Selected References
1. Haller J et al: Juxtaacetabular ganglionic (or synovial) cysts: CT and MR features. J Comput Assist Tomogr. 13:9/6, 1989
2. Li KC et al: MRI in osteoarthritis of the hip: Gradations of severity. Magn Res Imaging. 6:229,1988
3. Schurman DJ et al: Biochemistry and antigenicity of osteoarthritic and rheumatoid cartilage. J Orthop Res. 4:255, 1986

KNEE

Meniscal Radial Tear

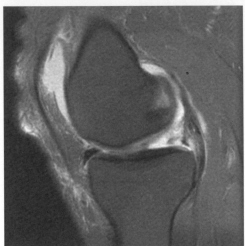

Radial tear of the medial meniscus involving the posterior horn.

Key Facts
- Vertical tear oriented perpendicular to the free edge of the meniscus
- May be degenerative or acute
- Associated with disruption of "hoop containment" when involving the posterior or anterior horn and allow subluxation of the body of the meniscus
- Posterior horn lateral meniscus radial tears associated with ACL tears

Imaging Findings
General Features
- Most commonly occurs at the junction of the anterior horn and body of the lateral meniscus and at the meniscotibial attachment of the posterior horn of the medial meniscus

MR Findings
- Increased signal intensity on short TE sequences within the free edge of the meniscus extending peripherally for a variable distance
- Often seen as blunting of the free edge on coronal images
- Often seen as diffuse, increased signal on one or two sagittal images next to normal or near normal meniscus on adjacent images due to tear orientation with respect to imaging plane

Differential Diagnosis
Horizontal Cleavage Tear
- Lacks vertical component
- Typically degenerative tear extending from the free edge apex horizontally into the meniscus

Oblique Meniscal Tear
- Usually contains horizontal component

Meniscal Radial Tear

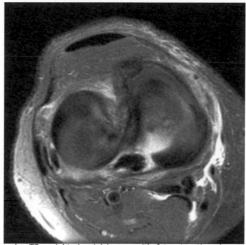

A fast spin echo T2 weighted axial image with fat saturation demonstrates high signal of the posterior horn of the medial meniscus giving a "Ghost like" appearance of the meniscus.

Other
- Bone trabecular injuries
- Chondral lesions
- Plica syndromes
- Ligament sprains

Pathology
General
- Etiology-Pathogenesis
  - Relatively uncommon meniscal tear
  - Usually develops insidiously in the lateral meniscus as a result of rotational forces acting across the meniscus at the "fulcrum" of movement between the spreading anterior and posterior horns during walking and running
  - Can occur acutely with a sudden impact

Gross Pathologic or Surgical Features
- Disruption of meniscal surface with a radial component (perpendicular to the longitudinal axis)
- May include displaced flap component

Microscopic Features
- Mucinous ground substance within the fibrocartilaginous meniscus with a separating cleavage plane surrounded by regenerative chondrocytes and fibrosis
- Variable degrees of synovial ingrowth
- Neovascularity in more chronic cases

Staging or Grading Criteria
- Tears of the meniscus represent grade III MRI signal abnormality
- Increased signal on short TE sequences extending to the articular surface

Meniscal Radial Tear

Clinical Issues
Presentation
- Adult
- Pain after single traumatic event or insidious onset of pain
- Joint line tenderness
- Feeling of "giving way"
- Clicking
- Locking if displaced fragment
- "Pseudolocking" if hamstring spasm is present

Treatment & Prognosis
- Debridement

Selected References
1. Stoller DW et al: The Knee, in Magnetic Resonance Imaging in Orthopaedics and Sports Medicine, D.W. Stoller, Editor. J.B. Lippincott: Philadelphia. 203-442, 1997
2. Jones RS et al: Direct measurement of hoop strains in the intact and torn human medial meniscus. Clin Biomech (Bristol, Avon). 11(5):295-300, 1996
3. Belzer JP et al: Meniscus Tears: Treatment in the Stable and Unstable Knee. J Am Acad Orthop Surg. 1(1):41-7, 1993

Meniscus Oblique Tear

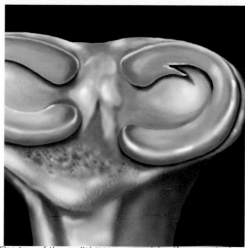

Flap tear of the medial meniscus involving the posterior horn.

Key Facts
- Obliquely oriented tear of the meniscus containing both longitudinal (long axis of meniscus) and radial (perpendicular to long axis) components
- Most common meniscal tear type
- Also called flap tear of the meniscus

Imaging Findings
General Features
- Most commonly affects posterior horn and is seen as predominantly horizontal on sagittal images originating along the inferior surface at the free edge
- May produce displaced flap
- Variable degrees of horizontal, vertical and radial components

MR Findings
- Obliquely oriented increased signal intensity on short TE sequences usually extending from the inferior surface on sagittal and coronal images
- May see fluid signal intensity on T2 weighted images
- Decreased signal intensity structure within the recess formed by the coronary ligament or meniscal femoral attachment in the case of a displaced flap (sequestered fragment)

Differential Diagnosis
Horizontal Cleavage Tear
- Lacks vertical component
- Typically degenerative tear extending from the free edge apex horizontally into the meniscus

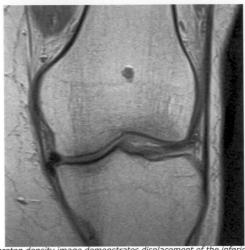

A coronal proton density image demonstrates displacement of the inferior leaf of the body of the medial meniscus into the recess formed by the coronary ligament.

<u>Other</u>
- Bone trabecular injuries
- Chondral lesions
- Plica syndromes
- Ligament sprains

Pathology
<u>General</u>
- Etiology-Pathogenesis
  - Most common meniscal tear
  - Can occur acutely with a sudden impact on the meniscus usually with a twisting component
  - May develop insidiously as a result of chronic shear forces across the meniscus

<u>Gross Pathologic or Surgical Features</u>
- Disruption of meniscal surface with a variable degree of longitudinal, radial and oblique components
- May include displaced flap component

<u>Microscopic Features</u>
- Mucinous ground substance within the fibrocartilaginous meniscus with a separating cleavage plane surrounded by regenerative chondrocytes and fibrosis
- Variable degrees of synovial ingrowth
- Neovascularity in more chronic cases

<u>Staging or Grading Criteria</u>
- Tears of the meniscus represent grade III MRI signal abnormality
  - Increased signal on short TE sequences extending to the articular surface

Meniscus Oblique Tear

Clinical Issues

<u>Presentation</u>
- Adult
- Pain after single traumatic event or insidious onset of pain
- Joint line tenderness
- Feeling of "giving way"
- Clicking
- Locking if displaced fragment
- "Pseudolocking" if hamstring spasm is present

<u>Treatment & Prognosis</u>
- Meniscal debridement/ partial meniscectomy

Selected References
1. Matava MJ et al: Magnetic resonance imaging as a tool to predict meniscal reparability. Am J Sports Med. 27(4):436-43, 1999
2. Stoller DW et al: The Knee, in Magnetic Resonance Imaging in Orthopaedics and Sports Medicine, D.W. Stoller, Editor. J.B. Lippincott: Philadelphia. 203-442, 1997
3. Belzer JP et al: Meniscus Tears: Treatment in the Stable and Unstable Knee. J Am Acad Orthop Surg. 1(1):41-7, 1993

Bucket Handle Meniscus Tear

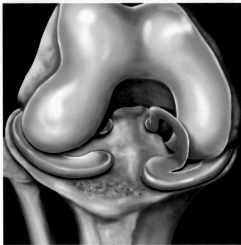

Bucket handle tear with displacement of medial meniscal tissue into the intercondylar notch.

Key Facts
- Displaced inner fragment of a vertical longitudinal tear of the meniscus
- Medial meniscus more common
- Typically an acute meniscal tear

Imaging Findings
General Features
- Displaced meniscus fragment resembles the handle of a bucket with the donor meniscus, still in place, representing the bucket itself
- Displaced fragment may be partially distracted or displaced all the way into the notch of the knee
- Displaced fragment may be attached to the donor meniscus at both ends or may be free at one end

MR Findings
- Coronal and sagittal images demonstrate blunting of the meniscus donor with the remaining meniscus being smaller than normal
- The "Double PCL Sign" represents the displaced fragment beneath the PCL at the notch of the knee resembling two PCL ligaments
- The "Double Delta Sign" represents a flipped inner meniscal fragment adjacent to the anterior horn of the donor meniscus producing two triangle shaped structures adjacent to each other

Differential Diagnosis
Oblique Intermeniscal Ligament
- Normal ligament extending from the anterior horn of the lateral meniscus to the posterior horn of the medial, vice versa or both mimicking a displaced fragment
- The menisci are normal in size without a recognizable donor site

Bucket Handle Meniscus Tear

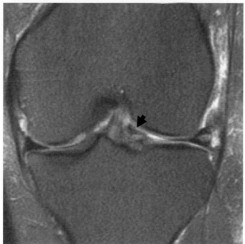

A coronal T2 weighted fast spin echo with fat saturation image demonstrates a bucket handle fragment (arrow) within the notch of the knee.

Scarred Chronic Disruption of the ACL
- Still only two structures in the notch (as in normal ACL and PCL) with one representing the scarred, decreased signal intensity torn displaced ACL

Pathology
General
- Etiology-Pathogenesis
  - o Relatively uncommon meniscal tear
  - o Usually occurs acutely with a sudden impact splitting the meniscus longitudinally
Gross Pathologic or Surgical Features
- Disruption of meniscal surface typically with a long longitudinal component involving the whole meniscus
Microscopic Features
- Mucinous ground substance within the fibrocartilaginous meniscus with a separating cleavage plane surrounded by regenerative chondrocytes and fibrosis
- Variable degrees of synovial ingrowth
- Neovascularity in more chronic cases
Staging or Grading Criteria
- Tears of the meniscus represent grade III MRI signal abnormality
- Increased signal on short TE sequences extending to the articular surface

Clinical Issues
Presentation
- Usually younger patient
- Pain after single traumatic event is typical
- Joint line tenderness
- Feeling of "giving way"

Bucket Handle Meniscus Tear

- Clicking
- Locking, typically a block preventing full extension

Treatment & Prognosis

- Repair if non displaced and affects the peripheral vascularized zone "red zone"
- Excision of fragment if tear extends through non vascularized free edge or if fragment is separated from parent meniscus

Selected References
1. Hame SL: Acute bucket-handle tear of the medial meniscus in a golfer. Arthroscopy. 17(6):E25, 2001
2. Elliott JM et al: MR appearances of the locked knee. Br J Radiol. 73(874):1120-6, 2000
3. Belzer JP et al: Meniscus Tears: Treatment in the Stable and Unstable Knee. J Am Acad Orthop Surg. 1(1):41-7, 1993

Discoid Meniscus

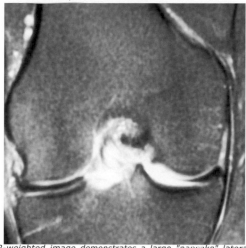

Coronal T2-weighted image demonstrates a large "pancake" lateral meniscus extending from the joint periphery to the intercondylar notch.

Key Facts
- Large, congenitally dysplastic meniscus with loss of the normal semilunar shape
- Lateral discoid meniscus is more common than medial discoid meniscus
- Sometimes bilateral

Imaging Findings
General Features
- Large or pancake-like meniscus
MR Findings
- Meniscal size greater than 13 mm in cross section is consistent with discoid morphology, normal: 5-13 mm from the capsular margin to the free edge on a central coronal image
- Meniscus exhibits continuous appearance of 3 consecutive sagittal 4-5 thick images
- Complete discoid meniscus has "pancake" appearance extending from the intercondylar notch to the periphery of the compartment
- Frequently demonstrates meniscal tear or intrameniscal tear seen as increased signal intensity on short TE images within the substance of the meniscus (intrameniscal tear) or extending to an articular surface (tear)
Plain Film Findings
- Widening of the joint space with hypoplastic femoral condyle and high fibular head in cases of lateral discoid meniscus
- Cupping of the lateral tibial plateau has been described

Differential Diagnosis
Any Condition Producing "Snapping Knee" Clinically
Patellofemoral Joint Subluxation
Meniscal Cysts

Discoid Meniscus

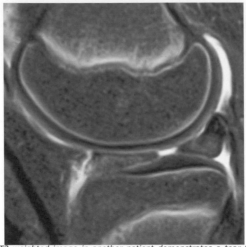

A sagittal T2-weighted image in another patient demonstrates a tear through the discoid meniscus.

<u>Vacuum Phenomenon</u>
- Typically in the hyperextended knee
- Decreased signal intensity in the joint between the weightbearing surfaces
- Rarely homogeneous like a discoid meniscus

<u>Flipped Meniscus</u>
- Meniscus is torn in this situation giving abnormal morphology to the "donor site" where portions of the meniscus are missing, thus allowing distinction from the discoid meniscus

Pathology

<u>General</u>
- Pancake or large meniscus which may demonstrate intrameniscal degeneration or meniscal tear

<u>Gross Pathologic or Surgical Features</u>
- Pancake or large, otherwise normal-appearing meniscus in the medial or lateral compartment
- Wrisberg-ligament type discoid meniscus lacks posterior capsular attachment

<u>Microscopic Features</u>
- Either microscopically normal meniscus or meniscus demonstrating mucoid chondral degeneration and/or tearing

<u>Staging or Grading Criteria</u>
- Watanabe classification
- Complete discoid meniscus extending into the intercondylar notch on coronal images
- Incomplete: Partially extends to the intercondylar notch on coronal images
- Wrisberg-ligament type: Lacks posterolateral meniscal tibial attachment

Discoid Meniscus

Clinical Issues

Presentation

- Congenital
- Patients often present with pain, clicking and snapping
- Locking is a common presentation in children
- Symptoms may not develop until adolescence or young adulthood
- Often asymptomatic

Treatment & Prognosis

- Partial meniscectomy with saucerization/partial resection of the discoid portion back to a more normal shaped meniscus

Selected References
1. Choi NH et al: Medial and lateral discoid meniscus in the same knee. Arthroscopy. 17(2):E9, 2001
2. Rohren EM et al: Discoid lateral meniscus and the frequency of meniscal tears. Skeletal Radiol. 30(6):316-20, 2001
3. Araki Y et al: MR imaging of meniscal tears with discoid lateral meniscus. Eur J Radiol. 27(2):153-60, 1998

Meniscal Cyst

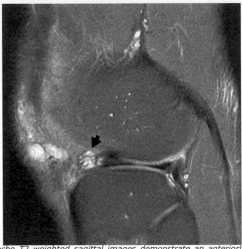

Fast spin echo T2 weighted sagittal images demonstrate an anteriorly dissecting parameniscal cyst (arrow). A meniscus tear was found at arthroscopy.

Key Facts
- Cyst that develops from the forcing of joint fluid into or through a meniscal tear, typically a horizontal tear
- More commonly involves the anterior horn of the lateral meniscus more than the posterior horn of the medial meniscus (2 most common locations)

Imaging Findings
General Features
- Cyst within (intrameniscal) or adjacent to (parameniscal) the meniscus typically in continuity with a meniscal tear
  - The meniscal tear is most commonly a horizontal cleavage tear off the posterior horn of the medial meniscus and anterior horn of the lateral meniscus and an oblique tear (radial at the free edge with horizontal extension into the periphery) at the junction of the body and posterior horn of the lateral meniscus

MR Findings
- Rounded, homogenous increased signal intensity mass on T2-weighted images which is intermediate to low signal intensity on T1-weighted images
- Mass sometimes lobulated and septated especially if parameniscal
- Cyst mass dissects around the knee into the paraarticular soft tissues
  - When medial the cyst dissects around the MCL or between the deep and superficial components
- If proteinaceous, the cyst may be of variable increased signal intensity on T1-weighted images

Differential Diagnosis
Synovial Cyst
- Doesn't originate from a meniscal tear

Meniscal Cyst

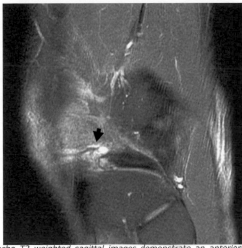

Fast spin echo T2 weighted sagittal images demonstrate an anteriorly dissecting parameniscal cyst (arrow). A meniscus tear was found at arthroscopy.

Bursitis
- Typically fluid within the semimembranosus or tibial collateral ligament bursa mimicking a medial parameniscal cyst. The deep infrapatellar bursa mimicking an anterior lateral parameniscal cyst with inferior extension

Cystic Masses
- Neoplastic masses tend to be heterogeneous with visible cellular elements

Pathology

General
- Etiology-Pathogenesis
  - Cyst arising from the extrusion of joint fluid through a meniscal tear often with a "ball valve" mechanism leading to a build up of pressure and cyst formation

Gross Pathologic or Surgical Features
- Cyst filled with mucinous, proteinaceous fluid within or adjacent to the meniscus in continuity with a horizontal cleavage meniscal tear or flap (oblique) tear with a predominately horizontal component

Microscopic Features
- Cyst formed within the meniscus lined by compressed meniscal collagen with variable areas of mucinous degeneration in the adjacent meniscus
- Cyst outside the meniscus (parameniscal) formed by compressed, paraarticular loose areolar tissue with variable degrees of hemorrhage and inflammatory cells

Clinical Issues

Presentation
- Adult patient
- Patient may present with pain and palpable mass near the joint line in cases of large cysts

Meniscal Cyst

- Cysts tend to be larger when lateral due to the loose soft-tissue constraints compared to the medial side

<u>Treatment & Prognosis</u>
- Resection of cyst and repair of tear

Selected References
1. Howell JR et al: Surgical treatment for meniscal injuries of the knee in adults. Cochrane Database Syst Rev. 2000
2. Rath E et al:The menisci: Basic science and advances in treatment. Br J Sports Med. 34(4):252-7, 2000
3. Stoller DW et al: The Knee, in Magnetic Resonance Imaging in Orthopaedics and Sports Medicine, D.W. Stoller, Editor. J.B. Lippincott: Philadelphia. 203-442, 1997

ACL Tear

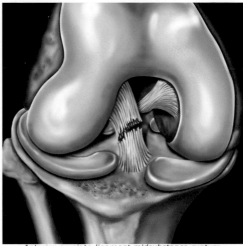

Anterior cruciate ligament midsubstance rupture.

Key Facts
- The most commonly disrupted ligament in the knee
- Tears are seen as disruption of the normal continuous decreased signal intensity ligament with irregularity and increased signal seen on T2 weighted MR images
- Tears are most commonly caused by forward translation of the tibia, external rotation of the femur with respect to the tibia, valgus stress and axial loading

Imaging Findings
General Features
- Disruption in the normal continuous linear ligament appearance
- Failure of ligament to parallel Blumensaat's line (intercondylar notch roof angle)
- Associated with bone trabecular injuries or impaction fractures of the posterolateral tibia and anterolateral femur
- Associated with meniscal tears (lateral greater than medial)
- Associated with posterolateral corner injuries (LCL, arcuate ligament, popliteus tendon, posterolateral capsule and other regional ligaments)

MR Findings
- Disruption of the normal linear decreased signal intensity ligament within the notch of the knee on all pulse sequences (sagittal and axial generally most helpful)
- Increased signal intensity disorganization and often thickening within the normally decreased signal intensity ligament best seen on T2-weighted images
- Axial T2-weighted images demonstrate thickening and increased signal intensity adjacent to the lateral intercondylar notch wall (normally the ligament is flat and decreased in signal intensity against the wall)
- Increased signal intensity with or without visible fracture lines or cortical impaction involving the posterolateral corner of the tibia, anterolateral femur and sometimes posterior medial tibia

ACL Tear

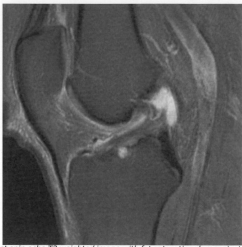

A sagittal fast spin echo T2 weighted image with fat saturation demonstrates horizontal orientation of the ACL with disruption of the proximal most fibers consistent with a tear.

- May see avulsion fracture of anterior tibial spine (especially in children)
- Buckling of the PCL on sagittal images due to forward translation of the tibia
- Hemorrhagic effusion common

Plain Film Findings
- Deepening of the anterolateral notch "lateral notch sign" (depression greater than 1.5 mm in depth at the condylopatellar sulcus)
- Segond fracture (avulsion of the meniscal tibial portion of the middle 3rd of the lateral capsular ligament)

Differential Diagnosis
Partial Tear
- May be difficult to diagnose on MRI
- See thickening, disruption of some fibers, abnormal orientation of some fibers
- Anteromedial bundle disruption more common than posterolateral bundle disruption in partial tears

Pathology
General
- Etiology-Pathogenesis: 3 common mechanisms of injury (anything that stresses the ligament and exceeds its capacity to maintain integrity)
  - Internal rotation, valgus stress, axial loading, forward translation of the tibia
    - Associated with posterolateral corner injury and antero-lateral femur injury
    - Seen with foot plant and subsequent external rotation of the thigh
  - Varus stress (sometimes associated with Segond fracture)
  - Hyperextension (uncommon)

ACL Tear

Gross Pathologic or Surgical Features
- Disruption of the ligament within its midsubstance, at its origin, or at its attachment accompanied by hemorrhage and synovitis (the latter finding in chronic cases)
- Avulsion of the anterior tibial spine seen especially in younger patients

Microscopic Features
- Disruption of normal collagen bundles accompanied by hemorrhage, various degrees of fibrosis, and inflammatory infiltration

Staging or Grading Criteria
- Partial tears (difficult to assess)
  - Less than 25% fiber disruption associated with more favorable prognosis
  - > 50% leads to insufficiency

Clinical Issues

Presentation
- Found in athletically active individuals most commonly
- Common injury in sports activities such as snow skiing, soccer, football, basketball, tennis and all sports characterized by rapid stopping, starting and pivoting
- Physical Examination Findings
  - Joint effusion in the acute case
  - Anterior drawer sign (forward translation of the tibia)
  - Lachman's sign (drawer test performed with 15 to 30 degrees knee flexion)
  - KTR arthrometer test for partial tears and associated laxity

Treatment & Prognosis
- ACL reconstruction in active patients

Selected References
1. Hawkins CA et al: ACL injuries in the skeletally immature patient. Bull Hosp Jt Dis. 59(4):227-31, 2000
2. Ho CP et al: MR imaging of knee anterior cruciate ligament and associated injuries in skiers. Magn Reson Imaging Clin N Am. 7(1):117-30, 1999
3. Stoller DW et al: The Knee, in Magnetic Resonance Imaging in Orthopaedics and Sports Medicine, D.W. Stoller, Editor. J.B. Lippincott: Philadelphia. 203-442, 1997

ACL Reconstruction

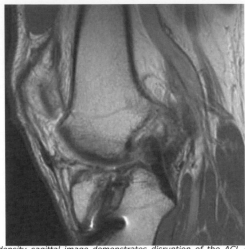

A proton density sagittal image demonstrates disruption of the ACL graft in this patient who is status post twisting injury.

Key Facts
- Bone-patellar tendon-bone and hamstring grafts are most commonly used intraarticular reconstructions
- Disruption of the graft results in discontinuous fibers within the notch associated with hemorrhage and generalized increased signal intensity on T2-weighted images

Imaging Findings
General Features
- Normal graft appears as linear decreased signal intensity structure paralleling the roof of the intercondylar notch (Blumensaat's line) on sagittal MR images
- The non-impinged graft (normal) is of decreased signal intensity on all pulse sequences with a large percentage of ligaments demonstrating intermediate signal intensity from 1 month to 6 months after grafting due to ligamentization and development of a synovial envelope

MR Findings
- The normal bone-patellar tendon-bone graft is of decreased signal intensity and parallels the intercondylar notch roof: A line drawn along the intercondylar notch roof (Blumensaat's line) should be continuous with the anterior wall of the tibial tunnel
- The hamstring graft (semitendinosus and gracilis tendons) may be associated with small amounts of fluid between the 2 components of the graft especially within the tibial or femoral tunnel
- Intermediate signal intensity from 6 weeks to 8 months is normally seen due to revascularization
- Roof impingement (forward placement of the tibial tunnel with resulting impingement of the intercondylar notch roof on the graft) results in increased signal intensity on all pulse sequences and variable disruption of fibers best seen on sagittal images

ACL Reconstruction

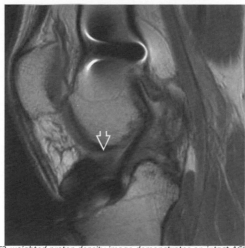

A sagittal T2-weighted proton density image demonstrates an intact ACL graft and a fibrous mass (arrow) immediately adjacent to Hoffa's fat pad consistent with a cyclops lesion.

- Graft disruption because of acute trauma is seen as discontinuous fibers and associated with meniscus tears, bony injuries and collateral ligament tears as with the native ACL
- Cyclops lesion - rounded decreased signal intensity mass (fibrotic) anterior to the graft may cause extension block and pain

Differential Diagnosis
Apparent Anterior Placement of Tibial Tunnel
- Forward translation of the tibia may result from graft disruption and tibial translation secondary to instability and not due to improper surgical placement

Revascularization
- Graft may exhibit intermediate signal intensity normally from 6 weeks to 8 months in the absence of roof impingement
- Important to have accurate history of surgery timing and presence of pain

Pathology
General
- Etiology-Pathogenesis
  - Most ACL reconstructions are currently intra-articular using either hamstring grafts or bone-patellar tendon-bone grafts
  - Abnormal placement of the tibial tunnel (usually anterior) can result in graft impingement

Gross Pathologic or Surgical Features
- Disrupted graft appears as discontinuous tendon fibers within the notch of the knee with variable degrees of hemorrhage and synovitis

Microscopic Features
- The tendon grafts progress through 4 stages of "ligamentization": Avascular necrosis, revascularization, cellular proliferation, and remodeling, resulting in histology closely resembling that of the native ACL
- Fibroblast healing occurs through the synovial membrane
- Revascularization occurs from the synovial membrane and endosteal vessels

Clinical Issues
Presentation
- Reconstruction goal is the maintenance of ligament isometric tension in order to keep the distance between the tibial and femoral attachment points from changing more than 2-3 mm through zero to 90° of flexion
- Graft placement depends upon activity level of the patients with active patients, in general, encouraged to have graft placed in order to prevent the development of osteoarthritis
- Roof impingement leads to pain and may eventually lead to graft disruption
  o Associated findings of impingement include: Joint effusion, decreased extension, pain, and recurrent instability
- Cyclops lesion may lead to pain and extension block
- Patellar tendonitis can occur at donor site (middle 3rd of patellar tendon)

Treatment
- Graft impingement treated with resection of osteophytes and replacement of graft if torn
- Cyclops lesion resected if symptomatic

Selected References
1. Jansson KA et al: MRI of anterior cruciate ligament repair with patellar and hamstring tendon autografts. Skeletal Radiol. 30(1):8-14, 2001
2. Veselko MA et al: Cyclops syndrome occurring after partial rupture of the anterior cruciate ligament not treated by surgical reconstruction. Arthroscopy. 16(3):328-31, 2000
3. Stoller DW et al: The Knee, in Magnetic Resonance Imaging in Orthopaedics and Sports Medicine, D.W. Stoller, Editor. J.B. Lippincott: Philadelphia. 203-442, 1997

PCL Tears

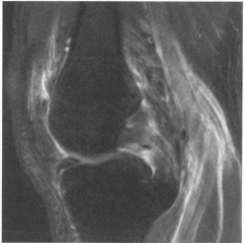

Fast spin echo T2 weighted sagittal image with fat saturation demonstrates disruption of the PCL.

Key Facts
- Accounts for only 5 to 20 percent of all knee ligament injuries (PCL is twice as strong as ACL)
- Most commonly occurs by direct trauma impacting the anterior knee in a posterior direction (dashboard injury)
- Most commonly diagnosed by imaging on MR images as discontinuous fibers and increased signal intensity on all pulse sequences

Imaging Findings
General Features
- Discontinuous and or thickened and increased signal intensity on all pulse sequences in the setting of trauma
- Posterior tibia insertion site avulsion fracture often seen
- Posterior lateral corner injury is associated

MR Findings
- Increased signal intensity on all pulse sequences is abnormal
- Normal ligament appears as decreased signal intensity "hockey stick" in the notch of the knee as seen on sagittal images
- Interstitial tear may appear as diffuse thickening and increased signal intensity
- Complete ruptures seen as increased signal intensity and discontinuous fibers on all pulse sequences
- Coronal images demonstrate thickening and increased intensity within the medial notch of the knee replacing the normal "hockey puck" appearance
- Avulsion fractures of the posterior mid tibia are well seen on all pulse sequences
- Anterior tibia bone trabecular injury or fracture and posterior femur injury may signify forced posterior displacement of tibia in a flexed knee

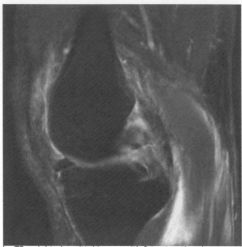

Fast spin echo T2 weighted sagittal image with fat saturation demonstrate disruption of the PCL.

- Increased signal intensity indicating bone injury of the anterior tibia and anterior femur "kissing fractures" are consistent with a hyperextension injury

Plain Film Findings
- Avulsion fractures of the posterior tibia seen
- Subtle anterior compaction fractures may be seen in some cases

Differential Diagnosis
Mucoid Degeneration
- Seen as a normal part of aging can lead to increased signal intensity and slight thickening

Pathology
General
- Etiology-Pathogenesis
  o Most commonly occurs as a dashboard injury but may also occur in hyperextension, dislocation and rotational injuries

Gross Pathologic or Surgical Features
- Disruption of the ligament within its midsubstance, at its origin, or at its attachment accompanied by hemorrhage and synovitis (the latter finding in chronic cases)

Microscopic Features
- Disruption of normal collagen bundles accompanied by hemorrhage, various degrees of fibrosis, and inflammatory infiltration

Clinical Issues
Presentation
- Can occur in children or adults and is the result of traumatic disruption
- Much less common than other ligament tears of the knee
- Positive posterior drawer sign (excessive mobility of the tibia posteriorly)

PCL Tears

- The posterior sagging sign is seen in complete tears where the tibia sags into a posterior subluxation relative to the femur with the patient supine and the knee flexed to 90 degrees
- The quadriceps active test results in translation of the tibia anteriorly during quadriceps contraction

Treatment & Prognosis
- Usually conservative
- Repair if a number of abnormalities present in association with ligament tear

Selected References
1.   Covey DC: Injuries of the posterolateral corner of the knee. J Bone Joint Surg Am. 83-A(1):106-18, 2001
2.   Fanelli GC: Treatment of combined anterior cruciate ligament-posterior cruciate ligament-lateral side injuries of the knee. Clin Sports Med. 19(3):493-502, 2000
3.   Stoller DW: The Knee, in Magnetic Resonance Imaging in Orthopaedics and Sports Medicine, D.W. Stoller, Editor. J.B. Lippincott: Philadelphia. 203-442, 1997

MCL Tear (Knee)

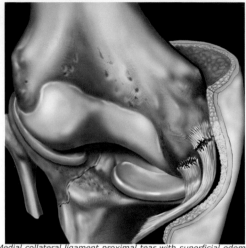

Medial collateral ligament proximal tear with superficial edema.

Key Facts
- Ligament disrupted by valgus stress on the knee which "opens up" the medial joint
- Associated injuries include ACL tears in injury to the peripheral aspect of the medial meniscus or meniscal attachments
- Disruption diagnosed as discontinuous ligament with thickening and increased signal intensity on all pulse sequences within the ligament remnant

Imaging Findings
General Features
- The superficial (tibial collateral ligament proper) and deep (meniscal femoral and meniscal tibial attachments) components can be disrupted completely or partially
- Calcification or ossification of the proximal ligament adjacent to the medial femoral epicondyle: Pellegrini-Stieda Disease is a chronic ligament sprain

MR Findings
- Increased signal within the ligament on T2-weighted images with fat saturation or STIR images
- Discontinuity of ligament fibers
- Heterotopic ossification (Pellegrini Stieda Disease) seen as increased signal (fat in bone marrow), corticated structure on T1 and proton density images
- Bone contusions involving the lateral femur and lateral tibia indicating valgus stress
- Partial tear: Some fibers are still continuous and intact

Differential Diagnosis
Osseous Injury
- Bone trabecular injuries medially or medial osteochondral injuries
Tibial Collateral Ligament Bursitis

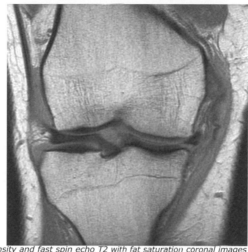

Proton density and fast spin echo T2 with fat saturation coronal images in a patient status post valgus stress injury demonstrates complete disruption of the MCI (grade 3).

Tibial Collateral Ligament Semimembranosus Bursitis
Medial Meniscus Tear

Pathology
General
- Etiology-Pathogenesis
  - Acute in valgus stress injury
  - Usually acute episode superimposed on chronic repetitive valgus stress
Gross Pathologic or Surgical Features
- Thickened, partially torn or completely torn ligament
Microscopic Features
- Degeneration, partial or complete rupture
- Variable amounts of hemorrhage and inflammatory cells
Staging or Grading Criteria
- Grade 1: Pain without instability, minimal tear
- Grade 2: Partial tear with some instability (50% or greater)
- Grade 3: Complete disruption

Clinical Issues
Presentation
- Child or adult after valgus injury physical examination findings include pain and instability (grade 2 and grade 3 sprains)
Treatment & Prognosis
- Isolated MCL sprains are treated with functional rehabilitation
- MCL sprains associated with ACL sprains are treated by repair of the ACL tear

MCL Tear (Knee)

Selected References
1. Woo SL et al: Healing and repair of ligament injuries in the knee. J Am Acad Orthop Surg. 8(6):364-72, 2000
2. Elliott JM et al: MR appearances of the locked knee. Br J Radiol. 73(874):1120-6, 2000
3. Stoller DW et al: The Knee, in Magnetic Resonance Imaging in Orthopaedics and Sports Medicine, D.W. Stoller, Editor. J.B. Lippincott: Philadelphia. 203-442, 1997

Posterolateral Complex Injury

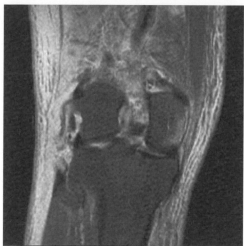

A STIR coronal T2 axial image demonstrates disruption of the fibular collateral ligament, popliteus tendon, arcuate ligament and other structures of the posterior lateral corner.

Key Facts
- The posterolateral (arcuate) complex includes the lateral collateral ligament, popliteus tendon, the lateral head of the gastrocnemius muscle, and the arcuate ligament
- Isolated lateral collateral ligament injury is less common than medial collateral ligament injury
- Associated with cruciate ligament tears
- Diagnosed as discontinuous ligament and or tendon fibers in association with edema in the posterolateral aspect of the knee

Imaging Findings
General Features
- Varus overload

MR Findings
- Increased signal intensity within the structures of the arcuate complex
- Fluid signal intensity within the ligaments and tendons in the case of a partial tear or complete tears
- Fast spin echo T2-weighted images with fat sat or STIR images demonstrate the increased signal to best advantage
- Avulsion of lateral tibia (Segond fracture)
- Fibular head avulsion fracture often seen

Differential Diagnosis
Lateral Meniscus Tear
- No injury to capsule, ligaments or tendons

Iliotibial Band Friction Syndrome
- Chronic fractional trauma between the iliotibial band and the lateral femoral condyle seen as increased signal intensity between the two structures on fat saturated T2 weighted images and variable thickening and increased signal intensity within the iliotibial band itself

Posterolateral Complex Injury

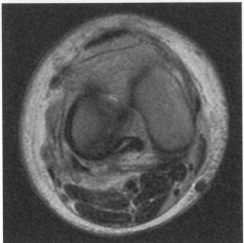

A fast spin echo T2 axial image demonstrates disruption of the fibular collateral ligament, popliteus tendon, arcuate ligament and other structures of the posterior lateral corner.

Pathology
General
- Etiology-Pathogenesis
  - The arcuate complex stabilizes the posterolateral aspect of the knee against varus stress and external rotation
  - With the leg in internal rotation valgus stress will lead to injury
  - A direct blow to the tibia with the knee flexed or extended or a twisting injury can result in cruciate ligament disruption and/or posterolateral instability
  - The fibular collateral ligament joins the tendon of the biceps femoris to form the conjoined tendon and it is rarely injured alone without injury to the remainder of the arcuate complex

Gross Pathologic or Surgical Features
- Tear of the structures of the arcuate complex with variable amounts of hemorrhage

Microscopic Features
- Microscopic and macroscopic tearing of the arcuate complex
- Variable amounts of hemorrhage and inflammatory cells

Clinical Issues
Presentation
- Post-traumatic abnormality seen in children and adults secondary to rotational mechanisms of injury described above
- Combined PCL and posterolateral capsular injuries are often missed at initial clinical presentation
- Injury characterized by posterolateral pain, buckling in hyper-extension with weight bearing and variable instability

Treatment & Prognosis
- Ligament and tendon disruptions are treated with repair
- If the cruciate ligament is damaged it is repaired

Selected References
1. Covey DC: Injuries of the posterolateral corner of the knee. J Bone Joint Surg Am. 83-A(1):106-18, 2001
2. Fanelli GC: Treatment of combined anterior cruciate ligament-posterior cruciate ligament-lateral side injuries of the knee. Clin Sports Med. 19(3):493-502, 2000
3. Ho CP et al: MR imaging of knee anterior cruciate ligament and associated injuries in skiers. Magn Reson Imaging Clin N Am. 7(1):117-30, 1999

Chondromalacia Patella

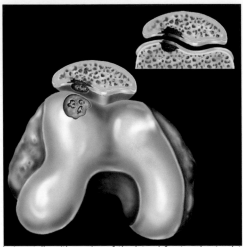

Chondromalacia patella with erosion of the lateral facet and anterolateral femoral condyle.

Key Facts
- Common cause of anterior knee pain
- Cartilage degeneration which begins as softening and progresses to fissuring or ulceration
- Most commonly degenerative in nature but can be acute and post-traumatic

Imaging Findings
General Features
- Fast spin echo proton density or T2 weighted MR images (especially with fat sat) or fat saturated spoiled gradient echo images are most useful

MR Findings
- Increased or decreased signal intensity on fat saturated fast spin echo images are seen in early changes
- Bone marrow and edema within the adjacent patella can signify acute changes (acute inflammatory chondromalacia) and/ or can signify ongoing stress versus a bone trabecular injury in cases of direct trauma
- Fissures or chondral defects often are seen in contrast to the adjacent fluid within the joint
- Subchondral cysts are seen in more chronic cases and often identified with full thickness chondral loss

Plain Film Findings
- Osteoarthritic changes are late findings and include osteophyte formation, subchondral cyst formation, bone attrition and remodeling, and subchondral sclerosis

Differential Diagnosis
Osteochondral Injuries of the Femoral Trochlea
- Hyaline articular cartilage abnormalities of the femoral trochlea with or without underlying bone changes in the presence of a normal patella

Chondromalacia Patella

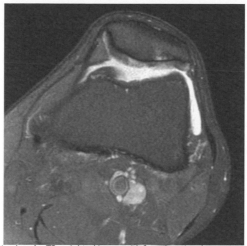

An axial fast spin echo T2 weighted image with fat saturation demonstrates increased signal intensity, partial thickness cartilage loss, surface irregularities and underlying bone edema consistent with chondromalacia patella. The cartilage abnormality is grade 2 to 3.

Patellar Tendinitis
* Increased signal intensity and/or thickening within the patellar tendon

Other
* Any other cause of anterior knee pain
* Anterior meniscal tears
* Inflammation of Hoffa's fat pad (hoffitis)
* Quadriceps tendinosis and/or tear

Pathology

General
* Etiology-Pathogenesis
  * Softening of the articular cartilage with associated degenerative changes including fissuring, chondral defects and underlying bone changes are all in the spectrum of patellofemoral chondromalacia
  * Patella alta, increased valgus angle, and femoral condyle hypoplasia predispose
  * Causes of acute chondromalacia include instability, direct trauma, and fracture
  * Causes of chronic chondromalacia include patellar subluxation, increased quadriceps angle (Q-angle), quadriceps imbalance, post-traumatic malalignment, excessive lateral pressure syndrome and PCL injuries

Gross Pathologic or Surgical Features
* Softening, discoloration, fissuring and or ulceration and desiccation

Microscopic Features
* Histologic changes of articular cartilage softening occur in the transitional zone deep to the superficial zone of articular cartilage and include reorientation and disorganization of collagen and fibers into collapsed segments associated with a decrease in matrix proteoglycans

Chondromalacia Patella

Staging or Grading Criteria
- Magnetic resonance imaging adaptation of Outerbridge arthroscopic grading system
- Grade 1
  - Fat suppressed T2-weighted fast spin echo images display focal areas of hyperintensity within normal contour
  - May include blistering
  - Softening by arthroscopy
- Grade 2
  - Fat suppressed T2-weighted fast spin echo images demonstrate fraying of the hyaline articular cartilage surface (crab meat by arthroscopy and MRI)
  - Fissuring and fibrillation within soft areas of the articular cartilage and extending to a depth of 1 to 2 mm within an area of 1.3 cm or less in diameter arthroscopically
- Grade 3
  - Fat suppressed T2-weighted fast spin echo images demonstrate partial thickness chondral defect
  - Partial thickness cartilage loss (> 2 mm depth in area and > 1.3 cm in diameter) arthroscopically
- Grade 4
  - Fat suppressed T2-weighted fast spin echo images demonstrate full thickness cartilage loss with underlying bone reactive changes
  - Full thickness chondral loss with exposed underlying bone (end-stage) arthroscopically

Clinical Issues
Presentation
- Most often affects adolescents and young adults
- May be characterized by insidious onset or acute and subsequent to patellar trauma
- Clinically characterized by patellofemoral joint pain, especially during flexion as can occur in ascending or descending stairs: Associated crepitus

Treatment & Prognosis
- Initial treatment is conservative and consists of rest and rehabilitation
- If instability is present surgical correction may be needed
- Direct surgical treatment of chondromalacia includes chondroplasty micro fracturing and chondral implantation

Selected References
1. Bosch JJ: Chondromalacia patella. J Pediatr Health Care. 13(3 Pt 1):144,155-6, 1999
2. Holmes SW: Clinical classification of patellofemoral pain and dysfunction. J Orthop Sports Phys Ther. 28(5):299-306, 1998
3. Van Leersum M et al: Chondromalacia patellae: an in vitro study. Comparison of MR criteria with histologic and macroscopic findings. Skeletal Radiol. 25(8):727-32, 1996

Patellar Tendinitis

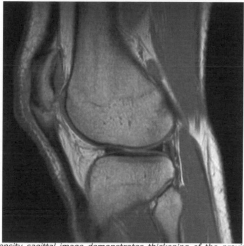

A proton density sagittal image demonstrates thickening of the proximal patellar tendon with a superimposed partial tear and surrounding edema.

Key Facts
- Chronic overuse tendinitis often due to sports containing jumping activities (jumper's knee)
- Most commonly affects the proximal 3rd of the patellar tendon
- MRI demonstrates thickening with or without partial or complete tearing and edema

Imaging Findings
General Features
- Findings are the general findings of tendinosis, partial tear and through-and-through tear

MR Findings
- Patellar tendinitis may demonstrate edema in the paratendon without visible change in the tendon itself
- Chronic tendinosis is characterized by thickening and areas of increased signal intensity (collagen degeneration) and/or decreased (normal) signal intensity indicating fibrosis
- Fluid signal intensity within the substance of the tendon or through the tendon is indicative of a partial tear or through-and-through tear respectively
- May see reactive edema within the lower pole of the patella (reactive osteitis)

Plain Film Findings
- May see thickening of the patellar tendon with edematous changes within Hoffa's fat pad

Differential Diagnosis
Pre-Patellar Bursitis (Housemaid's Knee)
- Localized fluid and inflammatory debris in the pre patellar bursa

Patellar Tendinitis

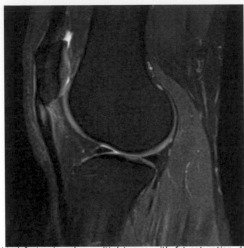

A T2-weighted fast spin echo sagittal image with fat saturation demonstrates thickening of the proximal patellar tendon with a superimposed partial tear and surrounding edema.

<u>Stress Response/Fracture of the Patella</u>
- Increased signal intensity with or without fracture lines in the presence of a normal patellar tendon

<u>Osgood-Schlatter's Disease</u>
- Imaging demonstrates osteochondrosis with variable hypertrophy of the tibial tuberosity and adjacent deep and/or superficial infrapatellar bursitis

<u>Sinding-Larsen-Johansson Disease</u>
- Osteochondrosis of the distal pole of the patella

<u>Other</u>
- Patellar sleeve avulsion fracture

Pathology

<u>General</u>
- Etiology-Pathogenesis
    - Degeneration, thickening and edema with collagen breakdown as results from chronic overuse commonly associated with jumping sports
    - Can occur in collagen vascular diseases along with tendinosis of other tendons
    - May occur acutely but usually in the setting of preexisting tendinosis

<u>Gross Pathologic or Surgical Features</u>
- Usually thickened indurated tendon
- Break in integrity of tendon in partially torn and torn tendons
- Partial tear may be proximal or distal

<u>Microscopic Features</u>
- Collagen degeneration without significant influx of inflammatory cells: "Tendinosis" is preferred term over tendinitis

Patellar Tendinitis

- Break in integrity of tendon in partially torn (bursal, articular or interstitial) and through-and-through torn tendons
- Fatty infiltration of muscle tissue in chronically torn tendons

Clinical Issues
Presentation
- Usually occurs in adults
- Malalignment of the extensor mechanism is contributory

Treatment & Prognosis
- Maquet's procedure of anterior tibial tubercle elevation results in a decrease in the forces that lead to overuse

Selected References
1. Duri ZA et al: Patellar tendonitis and anterior knee pain. Am J Knee Surg. 12(2):99-108, 1999
2. Verheyden FG et al: Jumper's knee: Results of surgical treatment. Acta Orthop Belg. 63(2):102-5, 1997
3. Stoller DW: The Knee, in Magnetic Resonance Imaging in Orthopaedics and Sports Medicine, D.W. Stoller, Editor. J.B. Lippincott: Philadelphia. 203-442, 1997

Pigmented Villonodular Synovitis

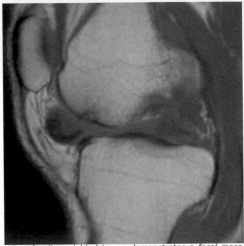

A sagittal proton density weighted image demonstrates a focal mass adjacent to Hoffa's fat pad representing the focal nodular form of pigmented villonodular synovitis (PVNS).

Key Facts
- Mono-articular synovial proliferative disorder
- Diffuse form and focal nodular form
- Images demonstrate hypertrophic synovium which is of variable but predominantly decreased signal intensity on all pulse sequences

Imaging Findings
General Features
- Diffusely thickened synovium which is of predominantly decreased signal intensity
- Focal nodular form typically found immediately adjacent to Hoffa's fat pad
- Gradient echo images demonstrate hemosiderin component to the best advantage due to blooming

MR Findings
- Diffusely thickened synovium with variable degrees of decreased signal intensity on all pulse sequences-diffuse form
- Focal mass typically immediately adjacent to the patella and/or Hoffa's fat pad of variable but generally decreased signal intensity on all pulse sequences

CT Findings
- CT arthrography demonstrates irregular and thickened synovium with or without erosions
- No calcification is demonstrated

Plain Film Findings
- Typically effusion is found
- Variable sized erosions with sclerotic margins may be found

Imaging Recommendations
- MRI is the most specific diagnostic tool

Pigmented Villonodular Synovitis

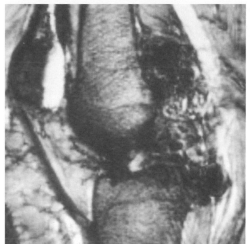

A sagittal T2* weighted image demonstrates thickened synovium which is of decreased signal intensity consistent with diffuse PVNS.

Differential Diagnosis
Hemophilic Arthropathy
- History is suggestive
- Almost always diffuse form

Hemorrhagic Synovitis
- Most commonly post-traumatic with appropriate history

Pathology
General
- Idiopathic mono-articular disorder

Gross Pathologic or Surgical Features
- Diffuse or focal hypertrophic synovitis containing blood breakdown products

Microscopic Features
- Hemosiderin laden macrophages within hyperplastic synovial masses often associated with sclerotic rimmed bone erosions
- Significant increase of chronic inflammatory infiltrates
- Characterized by proliferating mononuclear cells and fibroblasts activated by an excessive iron load
- Foam cells and giant cells are present

Clinical Issues
Presentation
- Mono-articular synovial disorder typically found and adults
- Nonpainful soft-tissue mass
- No sex predilection

Treatment & Prognosis
- Synovectomy

Selected References
1. Mancini GB et al: Localized pigmented villonodular synovitis of the knee. Arthroscopy. 14(5):532-6, 1998
2. Aigner TS et al: Iron deposits, cell populations and proliferative activity in pigmented villonodular synovitis of the knee joint. Verh Dtsch Ges Pathol. 82:327-31, 1998
3. Stoller DW et al: The Knee, in Magnetic Resonance Imaging in Orthopaedics and Sports Medicine, J.B. Lippincott:203-442, 1997

Osteochondritis Dissecans

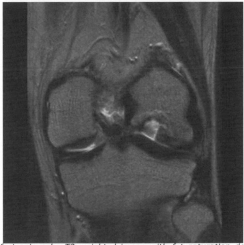

A coronal fast spin echo T2 weighted image with fat saturation demonstrates osteochondritis dissecans of the medial femoral condyle. Fluid undermines the fragment consistent with an unstable lesion.

Key Facts
- Osteochondrosis characterized by necrosis of bone followed by reossification and healing
- Usually affects the lateral aspect of the medial femoral condyle articular surface but can also affect the weight bearing surface of the lateral femoral condyle, tibia or patella
- Osteochondral abnormalities including a stable or unstable fragment characterizes the disease on MR Imaging
- A predisposing trauma history is found in approximately 50 percent of patients

Imaging Findings
General Features
- Osteochondral fragment of variable size either contiguous with the donor site or detached from it
- Predictors of instability include large size (greater than 1 cm), fluid interface between the fragment and donor site, cystic areas within the donor site, enhancement of granulation tissue on post gadolinium images between the donor site and fragment

MR Findings
- The focus of osteochondritis dissecans is seen as low signal intensity on T1 and T2-weighted images with variable amounts of edema both within the fragment and the adjacent donor site
- The overlying defects in the articular cartilage are best appreciated on fat suppressed T2-weighted fast spin echo or Stir images
- Fat saturated T2-weighted images may demonstrate direct extension of subchondral fluid indicating instability
- All pulse sequences may demonstrate loose osteochondral fragments
- Chondral fragments are best seen on fat saturated fast spin echo images

Osteochondritis Dissecans

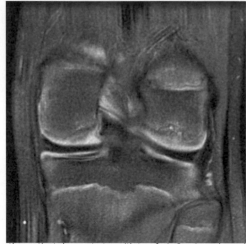

Another patient demonstrates with two foci: One in each condyle.

- MRI arthrography with intra-articular gadolinium may improve visualization of fluid across the articular cartilage surface thus helping determine whether the lesion is stable or unstable

Plain Film Findings
- May demonstrate an area of sclerosis typically affecting the lateral aspect of the medial femoral condyle with or without a loose fragment

Differential Diagnosis

Pathology

General
- Usually a lesion of adolescence often seen in athletes
- Unstable lesions
- Large size (typically greater than a centimeter)
- Cyst-like lesion beneath the osteochondrotic lesion
- Contains loose granulation tissue
- Loose fragment
  - Fluid insinuating beneath the fragment at arthrography
  - Loose body formation and residual deformity often present

Gross Pathologic or Surgical Features
- Necrotic desiccated bone fragment in unstable lesions

Microscopic Features
- Osteonecrosis with variable amounts of healing

Staging or Grading Criteria
- Based on arthroscopic findings
- Stage 1: The lesion is 1 to 3 cm in size with intact articular cartilage
- Stage 2: Articular cartilage defect without a loose body
- Stage 3: Partially detached osteochondral fragments with or without fibrous tissue interposition
- Stage 4: Loose body formation

Osteochondritis Dissecans

Clinical Issues

<u>Presentation</u>
- Primarily affects male patients 10 to 20 years of age often seen in athletes

<u>Treatment & Prognosis</u>
- Stable lesions treated with rest and splinting
- Unstable lesions often treated with abrasion chondroplasty, drilling or microfracture

Selected References
1. Sales de Gauzy JC et al: Natural course of osteochondritis dissecans in children. J Pediatr Orthop B. 8(1):26-8, 1999
2. Long G et al: Magnetic resonance imaging of injuries in the child athlete. Clin Radiol. 54(12):781-91, 1999
3. Cahill BR: Osteochondritis Dissecans of the Knee: Treatment of Juvenile and Adult Forms. J Am Acad Orthop Surg. 3(4) 237-47, 1995

Transient Patellar Dislocation

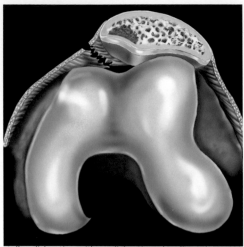

Transient patellar dislocation with medial retinacular disruption, contusion of the lateral aspect of the lateral femoral condyle and associated patellar facet contusion.

Key Facts
- Dislocation of the patella laterally as the result of a twisting injury with valgus stress or occasionally resulting from direct trauma
- Traumatic patellar dislocation occurs laterally
- Osteochondral injuries of the patella and lateral femoral condyle are common and associated with a tear of the medial retinaculum and/or a strain of the vastus medialis obliquus and disruption of the medial patellofemoral ligament
- Patella most often spontaneously reduces into the trochlear groove with extension following the injury

Imaging Findings
General Features
- Bone contusions of the anterior lateral femoral condyle and medial patella are diagnostic
MR Findings
- Osteochondral injuries of the patella and lateral femoral condyle are common and associated with a tear of the medial retinaculum and/or a strain of the vastus medialis obliquus and disruption of the medial patellofemoral ligament
- Disruption of the origin of the medial patellofemoral ligament is seen as increased signal intensity at the junction of the medial collateral ligament and the medial patellofemoral ligament best seen on fat saturated fast spin echo T2-weighted images in the axial plane
    - Disruption of this ligament is often surgically treated
- Hemarthrosis is seen as fluid signal intensity on T2-weighted images with variable amounts of decreased signal intensity, debris, and sometimes a fluid-fluid level
- Chondral or osteochondral fragments may be free floating within an effusion and are important to identify: Lateral patellar tilt or subluxation may be seen

Transient Patellar Dislocation

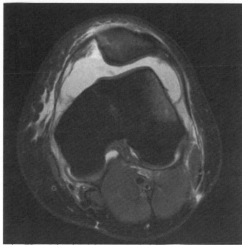

A fast spin echo T2-weighted axial image with fat saturation demonstrates a bone trabecular injury of the medial patella and anterior lateral femoral condyle. A pattern consistent with a recent patellar dislocation.

Plain Film Findings
- A fracture of the patella or anterior lateral femoral condyle may be found

Differential Diagnosis
ACL Tear with Hemarthrosis
- May mimic a transient patellar dislocation clinically
Osteochondral Injury Anteriorly without Patellar Dislocation

Pathology
General
- Etiology-Pathogenesis
  - May occur secondary to a shallow trochlear groove, ligamentous laxity or both
  - Abnormal iliotibial band and vastus lateralis attachment may produce a lateral patellar pull
  - Intrinsic muscle abnormalities and soft-tissue damage may predispose to dislocation
  - Variation of patellar shapes (Weiberg types) may predispose to dislocations including type 3 (small and convex medial patellar facet) and type 5 (Jägerhut or hunter's cap) patella: Patella alta with subsequent loss of containment by the lateral femoral condyle predisposes to dislocations
Gross Pathologic or Surgical Features
- Osteochondral injuries of the patella and lateral femoral condyle are common and associated with a tear of the medial retinaculum and/or a strain of the vastus medialis obliquus and disruption of the medial patellofemoral ligament

<u>Microscopic Features</u>
- Findings are those of fracture and ligamentous disruption and chondral injury

Clinical Issues
<u>Presentation</u>
- May occur in childhood especially in patients with congenitally shallow trochlear groove but occurs throughout adulthood secondary debt twisting injury, valgus stress or direct blow

<u>Treatment & Prognosis</u>
- Non operative treatment includes cast immobilization and rehabilitation with early return of range of motion and strength
- Arthroscopy is used in the diagnosis and treatment of osteochondral fragments and associated intra articular pathology as well as performing selective lateral retinacular release: Lateral retinacular release relieves the retinacular pull

Selected References
1. Carrillon YH et al: Patellar instability: Assessment on MR images by measuring the lateral trochlear inclination-initial experience. Radiology. 216(2):582-5, 2000
2. Nomura E: Classification of lesions of the medial patello-femoral ligament in patellar dislocation. Int Orthop. 23(5):260-3, 1999
3. Holmes SW et al: Clinical classification of patellofemoral pain and dysfunction. J Orthop Sports Phys Ther. 28(5):299-306, 1998

PocketRadiologist™
Musculoskeletal
100 Top Diagnoses

ANKLE AND FOOT

Achilles Tendon Tear

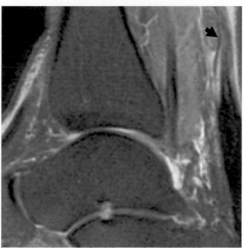

Complete rupture (arrow) of Achilles tendon (FST2-FSE sagittal image).

Key Facts
- Athletic activity in middle-aged males
- Direct trauma: Rupture at the myotendinous junction
- Rupture 2-6 cm superior to the os calcis

Imaging Findings
MR Findings
- Normal Achilles tendon is of uniform hypointensity
- Rupture/tear = disruption with discontinuity +/- wavy retracted tendon
- T1 and FST2-FSE or STIR sagittal and axial images required
- Hyperintense hemorrhage or edema on FST2-FSE images in intratendinous or peritendinous soft tissue
- Hyperintense fluid-filled gap +/- interposed fat
- Proximal tendon retraction associated with fraying or corkscrewing of tendon edges
- Intratendinous fluid: May be seen up to six months postsurgical treatment or conservative management (a widened tendon up to 12 months)
- Enlarged proximal and distal ends may be associated with an attenuated union bridging the tear site
- Surgical repair healing response: Increased size of tendon associated with decreased tendinous signal intensity secondary to scar tissue
- Associated edema in peritenon and preachilles fat is a common finding

Differential Diagnosis
Partial Tear of the Achilles Tendon
- Without tendinous gap

Plantaris Tendon Tear
- A torn plantaris tendon may mimic an Achilles tendon tear on medial sagittal images (an intact plantaris tendon may also be seen in the presence of an Achilles tendon rupture)

Achilles Tendon Tear

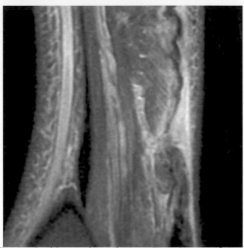

Corresponding proximal image shows the tear site and extent of proximal tendon retraction (FST2-FSE sagittal image).

Pathology

<u>General</u>
- Etiology-Pathogenesis
  - Forced dorsiflexion of foot against contracting force (triceps surae group)
  - Rheumatoid arthritis, systemic lupus, diabetes mellitus and gout
  - Acute rupture: Predisposing factors include chronic tendinitis and partial tears

Clinical Issues

<u>Presentation</u>
- Pain and soft-tissue swelling (hemorrhage)
- Clinical assessment can be missed up to 25% of cases
- Thompson test positive if squeezing calf did not produce plantar flexion response
- MR imaging identifies tendinous gap important for conservative management (retracted tendons are less likely to heal with large diastasis)

<u>Treatment & Prognosis</u>
- Surgical repair usually required
- Recurrent rupture
  - 10 to 30% with conservative treatment
  - 5% with surgical treatment

Selected References
1. Dillon E et al: Achilles tendon healing: 12-month follow up with MR imaging. Radiology. 177P: 306, 1990
2. Keene JS et al: Magnetic resonance imaging of Achilles tendon ruptures. Am J Sports Med. 17:333, 1989
3. Quinn SP et al: Achilles tendon: MR imaging at 1.5 T. Radiology. 164:767, 1987

Osteochondral Lesion of Talus

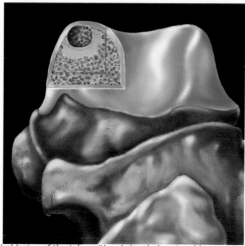

Osteochondral lesion of the talus with subchondral cyst and bone marrow edema of the talus.

Key Facts
- Osteochondral leasion of the talus (OLT), transchondral fracture, osteochondral fracture, osteochondritis dissecans and talar dome fracture are equivalent terms
- Involve articular cartilage and subchondral bone medial (60%) and lateral (40%)
- Antecedent trauma (e.g. torsional impaction)
- Chronic phase of compressed or avulsed talar dome fracture

Imaging Findings
Plain Film & CT Findings
- May be insensitive to early or occult OLT (Stage I)
- Cannot access integrity of hyaline articular cartilage
MR Findings
- Four stage MR classification
  - Stage I: Subchondral trabecular compression with marrow edema
  - Stage IIA: Subchondral cyst
  - Stage IIB: Incomplete separation of fragment
  - Stage III: Fluid around undetached, undisplaced fragment
  - Stage IV: Displaced fragment
- Normal articular cartilage: Intermediate signal intensity using FST2-FSE
- Detached cortical fragment: Hypointense
- Bony defect: Hypointense to intermediate on T1-weighted images (as a function of fluid and fibrous tissue)
- Fluid: Hyperintense on T2-weighted images
- Reactive bone sclerosis: Peripheral hypointensity on T1 and T2-weighted images
- Adjacent subchondral talar marrow edema
  - Extends beyond focus of necrosis
  - Hyperintense on FST2-FSE and STIR images
- Chondral abnormalities, thinning, upward bowing, nodularity, and disruption (including flap lesions)

Osteochondral Lesion of Talus

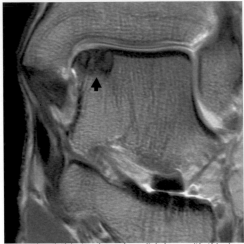

Hypointense osteochondral lesion (arrow) medial dome with thinning of overlying subchondral plate and articular cartilage (T1-weighted coronal image).

- Chondral fissures and defects: Focal hyperintensity or undermining fluid
- Postsurgical fibrocartilaginous scar: Intermediate signal intensity bridging defect
- FST2-FSE and STIR images more sensitive than T2* weighted images for articular cartilage
- Partially attached fragment: Irregular, hyperintense zone at fragment, talar interface
- Unattached fragment: Complete ring of hyperintense fluid on FST2-FSE or STIR images
- Granulation tissue: Increased signal at fragment subchondral bone interface without chondral violation
- Intravenous MR contrast: Evaluate congruity of articular cartilage, enhance subchondral edema and synovial tissue
- Intraarticular contrast: For unstable and free fragment evaluation (not routinely used)

Differential Diagnosis
Degenerative Sclerosis
- Usually involves tibial and talar surfaces
AVN
- May show a more diffuse pattern of talar edema compared to OLT

Pathology
General
- Etiology-Pathogenesis
  - Direct trauma or repetitive microtrauma
  - Osteonecrotic process leads to subchondral fracture and collapse
  - Synovial fluid influxed and increased joint pressure: Prevents healing
  - Forced inversion and dorsiflexion: Lateral lesions in mid to anterior talar dome

- o Forced inversion and plantar flexion with external rotation: Medial lesion

<u>Staging or Grading Criteria</u>
- Berndt and Harty four-part staging based on conventional radiographs

Clinical Issues
<u>Presentation</u>
- Antecedent trauma (e.g. torsional impaction)
- Delayed diagnosis: Leads to arthritis in 50% of cases
- Medial lesions: Cup shaped and deeper
- Lateral lesions: Wafer shaped or thin (antecedent trauma)

<u>Treatment & Prognosis</u>
- Based on stage and acute vs chronic
  - o Stage I and II: Immobilization
  - o Stage III or IV: Free fragment excision, curettage, drilling or abrasion arthroplasty
- Complication: Degenerative arthritis

Selected References
1. Ferkel RD et al: Arthroscopic treatment of osteochondral lesions of the talus: Long-term results, Orthop Trans. 17:1011, 1993-4
2. De Smet AA et al: Value of MR imaging in staging osteochondral lesions of the talus (osteochondritis dissecans): Results in patient. AJR.154: 555, 1990
3. Yulish BS et al: MR imaging of osteochondral lesions of the talus. J Comput Assist Tomogr. 1:296, 1987

Tibialis Posterior Tendon Tear

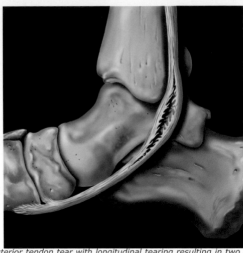

Tibialis posterior tendon tear with longitudinal tearing resulting in two subtendons.

Key Facts
- Spontaneous or with associated synovitis, steroid injection or trauma
- Chronic rupture in middle aged women in fifth or sixth decades
- Unilateral flatfoot deformity without history of trauma
- Spectrum of degeneration and longitudinal splitting on MR images
- Site of rupture within 6 cm proximal to navicular insertion
- Osteophytic spur of medial malleolus

Imaging Findings
MR Findings
- Complete tears: Disruption +/- abnormal morphology of tendon ends
- Partial, chronic tear or retracted tendon: Associated with enlargement of tendon on cross-sectional diameter
- Tenosynovitis: Seen in tears and degeneration as hyperintense fluid on FST2-FSE and STIR images
- Type I tear: Tendon hypertrophy with heterogeneous (increased signal intensity on T1 and FST2-FSE) signal intensity in vertical split
- Type II tears: Attenuated section of tendon at level of medial malleolus
- Type III tear: Complete with tendinous gap
- Subtendons seen in Type I and Type II tears
- Associated findings: Hypertrophy medial tubercle navicular, abnormal talonavicular alignment, accessory navicular
- Chronic dysfunction: Spring ligament laxity or rupture

Differential Diagnosis
Tendinosis
- Intrasubstance degeneration without longitudinal splitting or increased axial diameter

Tenosynovitis
- Tendon morphology is maintained

Tibialis Posterior Tendon Tear

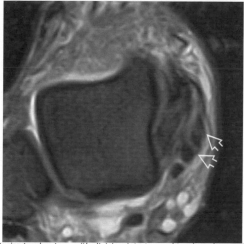

Tibialis posterior tendon tear with division into two subtendons (arrows) anterior to the flexor digitorum longus (FST2-FSE axial image).

Pathology
General
- Etiology-Pathogenesis
  - Intrinsic degeneration of tendon
  - Spontaneous rupture (excluding rheumatoid involvement): Tibialis posterior muscle fatigue against pronation, vulnerable blood supply, acute angulation of tendon posterior to medial malleolus, pes planovalgus

Clinical Issues
Presentation
- Unilateral involvement 90%
- Medial pain, swelling and tenderness
- Collapse of medial longitudinal arch: Flatfoot deformity + heel valgus, talar plantar flexion and forefoot abduction
- Forefoot abduction: Associated lateral subluxation navicular
- Weakness of inversion

Treatment & Prognosis
- Support medial longitudinal arch, surgical debridement, osseous stabilization (arthrodesis) or repair
- Side-to-side anastomosis to flexor digitorum longus

Selected References
1. Karasick D et al: Tear of the posterior tibial tendon causing asymmetric flatfoot: Radiologic findings. AJR. 161:1237, 1993
2. Schweitzer ME et al: Posterior tibial tendon tears: Utility of secondary signs for MR imaging diagnosis. Radiology. 188:655, 1993
3. Rosenberg ZS et al: Rupture of posterior tibial tendon: CT and MR imaging with surgical correlation. Radiology. 169:229, 1988

Tibialis Anterior Tendon Tear

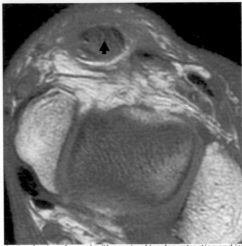

Tibialis anterior tendon tear (arrow) with proximal tendon retraction and intrasubstance degeneration (T1-weighted axial image).

Key Facts
- Rupture between extensor retinaculum and insertion onto medial first cuneiform and adjacent base first metatarsal
- Weakness dorsiflexion, local tenderness and drop-foot gait
- Spontaneous rupture rare < 50 years of age
- Acute ruptures in athletes: Forced plantar flexion and ankle eversion

Imaging Findings
MR Findings
- Oblique axial images perpendicular to tendon at level of medial malleolus
- Partial tear: Focal enlargement with hyperintense split on FST2-FSE or gadolinium contrast enhanced image
- Complete rupture: Fluid-filled gap hyperintense on FST2-FSE images and partial proximal retraction
- Oblique coronal images parallel to long axis

Differential Diagnosis
Partial Tear Versus Complete Tear
- Axial oblique and coronal oblique images required

Pathology
General
- General Path Comments
  - Blood supply exclusive from the anterior tibial artery – tendon at risk for ischemia
  - Rupture between superior and inferior extensor retinaculum and medial tarsometatarsal joint (dorsal osteophyte)
- Etiology-Pathogenesis
  - Degenerative-spontaneous vs trauma with plantar flexion vs direct laceration

Tibialis Anterior Tendon Tear

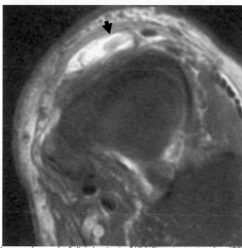

Complete absence (arrow) of distal extent of tibialis anterior tendon (FST2-FSE axial image).

Clinical Issues
Presentation
- Footdrop
- Palpable mass secondary to retracted proximal tendon superior to inferior retinaculum

Treatment & Prognosis
- Conservative vs repair in complete ruptures

Selected References
1. Khoury NJ et al: Rupture of the anterior tibial tendon: Diagnosis by MR imaging. AJR. 167:351, 1996
2. Ouzounian TJ et al: Anterior tibial tendon rupture. Foot Ankle. 16:406, 1995

Peroneus Brevis Tendon Tear

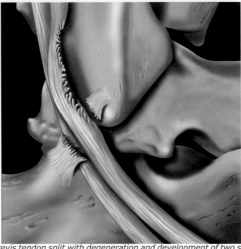

Peroneus brevis tendon split with degeneration and development of two sub-tendons.

Key Facts
- Rupture secondary to trauma or laceration
- Partial tear: Split more common than complete tear
- Preexisting tendon degeneration
- Spontaneous rupture: Brevis more common than longus

Imaging Findings
MR Findings
- Longitudinal splits: Best shown on axial images (secondary visualization on coronal and sagittal planes)
- Tendinosis: With either tendon thickening or attenuation
- Fluid hyperintense in association with tenosynovitis
- Tears: Level of lateral malleolus
- Associated sprain of superior retinaculum or lateral ligament complex
- Complete rupture: Reactive calcaneal marrow edema at lateral attachment of inferior peroneal retinaculum (peroneal tubercle)
- Fibular groove: Roughening or osteophyte in posterolateral aspect of fibula
- Peroneus longus tendon: May interpose between the two subtendons of brevis

Differential Diagnosis
Tendinosis
- Partial tear with discrete, linear, hyperintense signal intensity (intrasubstance signal)
  - No subtendons

Pathology
General
- Etiology-Pathogenesis
  - Rupture secondary to trauma or laceration

Peroneus Brevis Tendon Tear

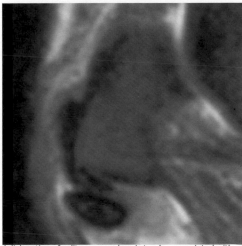

Anterolateral dislocation of split peroneus brevis tendon associated with a torn superior peroneal retinaculum (FST2-FSE axial image).

- o   Preexisting tendon degeneration
- • General Path Comments
  - o   Longitudinal splits plus hypertrophy (two subtendons = peroneal split syndrome)
  - o   CF (calcaneal fibular) ligament or fibular lateral cartilaginous ridge: Abrasion of brevis in development of longitudinal tears
  - o   Lateral ligament tears + laxity superior peroneal retinaculum lead to peroneus brevis split and peroneal tendon subluxation
  - o   Calcaneal fractures associated with entrapment or tear

Clinical Issues

Presentation
- • Acute injury or spontaneous presentation
- • Peroneal tendons = lateral stabilizers of the ankle
- • Brevis important to eversion of the foot

Treatment & Prognosis
- • Debridement of split

Selected References
1.   Khoury NJ et al: Peroneus longus and brevis tendon tears: MR imaging evaluation. Radiology. 200:833, 1996
2.   Geppert MJ et al: Lateral ankle instability as a cause of superior peroneal rednacular laxity: An anatomic and biomechanical study of cadaveric feet. Foot Ankle. 14:330, 1993

ATFL Tear

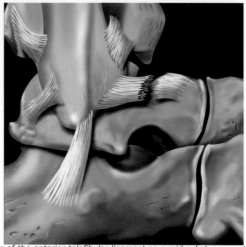

Tear of the anterior talofibular ligament as a mid substance rupture.

Key Facts
- Inversion and internal rotation combined with plantar flexion
- Anterior talofibular ligament tear (ATFL) restrains internal rotation
- Weakest of lateral ligaments and first to rupture
- Anterior displacement of talus
- Tear of ATFL + CFL = widening of lateral joint space and medial tilt of talus

Imaging Findings
MR Findings
- ATFL identified on axial images coursing in a 45-degree angle from lateral malleolus to talus
- Associated capsule rupture + extension of fluid anterolaterally into soft tissues
- Acute tears associated with partial ligament disruption, ligament laxity or complete absence of ligament
- Adjacent hemosiderin or edema identified
- Medial talar bone contusion hyperintense on FST2-FSE images
- Avulsed ligament +/- distal fibular avulsion fracture

Differential Diagnosis
Synovitis
- Excessive plantar flexion obscures ligament visualization on axial images
Sprain
- No ligamentous discontinuity (requires FST2-FSE images)

Pathology
General
- Etiology-Pathogenesis
  - Inversion and internal rotation combined with plantar flexion

ATFL Tear

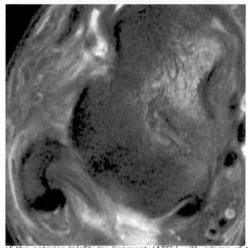

Acute tear of the anterior talofibular ligament (ATFL) with edema of the anterior aspect of the lateral gutter (FST2-FSE axial image).

Staging or Grading Criteria
- Grade I: Stretching and partial tear
- Grade II: Moderate sprain with edema and partial tear of ATFL and CFL
- Grade III: Complete tear of ATFL and CFL with ankle instability

Clinical Issues
Presentation
- Chronic tears associated with meniscoid lesion (interposed between talus and fibula)
- Subtalar arthrosis
- Complication: Anterolateral impingement

Treatment & Prognosis
- Conservative
- Surgery: Associated OLT (osteochondral lesion of the talus)
- Broström procedure: Suturing
- Modified Broström: Capsular shift
- Chrisman-Snook procedure: Tenodesis of peroneus brevis tendon
- Watson-Jones procedure: Tenodesis of peroneus brevis

Selected References
1. Colville MR: Reconstruction of the lateral ankle ligaments. J Bone Joint Surg [Am]. 76A: 1092, 1994
2. Rijke et al: MRI of lateral ankle ligament injuries. Am J Sports Med. 21:527, 1993
3. Erickson SJ et al: MR imaging of the lateral collateral ligament of the ankle. AJR. 156:131, 1991

Deltoid Ligament

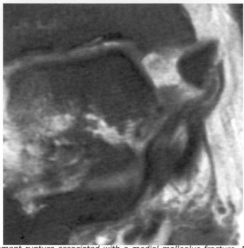

Deltoid ligament rupture associated with a medial malleolus fracture. No tibiotalar fibers are identified. Lateral compartment contusions are associated (FST2-FSE coronal image).

Key Facts
- Sprains more common than complete tear
- Partial tears associated with inflammatory or edematous changes
- Osseous avulsions visualized on coronal and sagittal images through mid medial malleolus
- Isolated injuries rare

Imaging Findings
General Features
- Tears as either interstitial or avulsion
- Complete tear: Superficial and deep layers seen with fracture of lateral malleolus
- Talar displacement laterally or posterolaterally

MR Findings
- Diffuse/amorphous hyperintensity on FST2-FSE images
- Indistinct margins and loss of fiber striation (tibiotalar fibers) on FST2-FSE
- Axial and coronal images best for separating superficial from deep layer injuries
- Mass-like morphology: Complete disruption + edema, hemorrhage and granulation tissue
- Gadolinium enhancement: Useful in showing partial tears

Differential Diagnosis
Normal Tibiotalar Ligament
- With interposed fatty tissue
- Partial volume of periligamentous fatty or fibrocartilaginous tissue

Deltoid Ligament

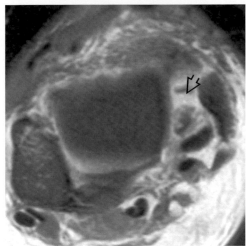

Corresponding axial plane image shows a fluid-filled gap (arrow) replacing superficial and deep layers of the deltoid ligament (FST2-FSE axial image).

Pathology

General
- General Path Comments
  - Superficial layer
    - Superficial anterior tibiotalar
    - Tibionavicular
    - Tibioligamentous
    - Tibiocalcaneal
    - Superficial posterior tibiotalar
  - Deep layer
    - Small anterior component: Anterior talotibial
    - Strong posterior talotibial ligament
- Etiology-Pathogenesis
  - Eversion also endstage of supination external rotation injuries

Staging or Grading Criteria
- Grade I: Hyperintensity, thickening and subcutaneous edema
- Grade II: 50% ligament disruption with hyperintensity +/- focal fluid and ligamentous thickening
- Grade III: Hyperintense fluid-filled gap or absent ligament

Clinical Issues

Presentation
- Associated lateral ligamentous injury, fibular fracture and/or syndesmosis injuries
- Widened ankle mortise more common with deltoid injuries in association with preexisting lateral complex pathology

Treatment & Prognosis
- Conservative vs debridement and repair in unstable tibiotalar joints

Deltoid Ligament

Selected References
1.   Klein MA: MR imaging of the ankle: normal and abnormal findings in the medial collateral ligament. AJR. 162:377, 1994
2.   Chandnani VP et al: Chronic ankle instability: evaluation with MR arthrography, MR imaging and stress radiography. Radiology. 192:189, 1994

Syndesmosis Sprain

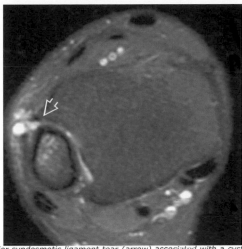

Anterior syndesmotic ligament tear (arrow) associated with a cystic fluid collection.

Key Facts
- Ligaments: Anterior inferior tibiofibular (AITF), posterior inferior tibiofibular (PITF), the transverse tibiofibular ligament and the interosseous membrane
- External rotation is primary mechanism
- AITF more common than PITF injury
- Syndesmosis sprain: 10% of all ankle injuries

Imaging Findings
MR Findings
- Ligament thickening: Increase anterior to posterior dimension of either the anterior or posterior syndesmotic ligament + intraligamentous hyperintensity
- Contour irregularity of the syndesmotic ligament (AITF or PITF)
- Frank discontinuity of ligament
- Intraosseous membrane injury: Linear hyperintensity on FST2-FSE or STIR at level of distal tibia and fibula between AITF and PITF
- Hyperintense foci in interosseous membrane = hemosiderin, fibrosis or calcification
- Diastasis of tibiofibular joint

Differential Diagnosis
Synovitis
- Without ligament hyperintensity, laxity or discontinuity

Pathology
General
- Etiology-Pathogenesis
  - External rotation and hyperdorsiflexion
  - Transverse tibiofibular ligament forms true posterior labrum

Syndesmosis Sprain

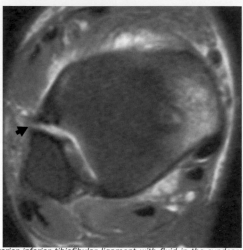

Tear of anterior inferior tibiofibular ligament with fluid in the syndesmosis. Medial malleolus bone contusion is present (FST2-FSE axial image).

Clinical Issues
Presentation
- Acute swelling is uncommon
- Football and downhill skiing injuries
- Syndesmotic impingement as a complication
  - Inflamed synovium (synovial nodules)
  - Scarring of AITF
  - Loose bodies, chondromalacia and osteophytes
  - Abrading of lateral talar dome: Separate fascicle of AITF

Treatment & Prognosis
- Conversative unless unstable syndesmosis

Selected References
1. Ogilvie-Harris DJ et al: Disruption of the ankle syndesmosis: Diagnosis and treatment by arthroscopic surgery. Arthroscopy. 10:561, 1994
2. Schneck CD et al: MR imaging of the most commonly injured ankle ligaments, I. Normal anatomy. Radiology. 184:499, 1992

Sinus Tarsi Syndrome

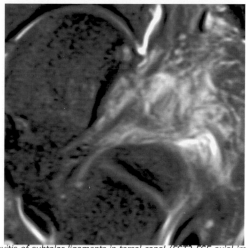

Synovitis of subtalar ligaments in tarsal canal (FST2-FSE axial image).

Key Facts
- Lateral foot pain and tenderness
- Subtalar microinstability
- Frank ankle instability not present
- 60% of patients with abnormal tarsal sinus and canal on MRI

Imaging Findings
MR Findings
- Tears of the sinus tarsi ligaments
- Fibrosis of sinus tarsi ligaments (hypointense on T1 and T2)
- Synovitis, fluid and sprain of ligaments hypointense on T1 and hyperintense on T2 (FST2-FSE and STIR images)
- Hyperintensity of fluid in anterior and posterior microrecesses at posterior facet subtalar joint (T2 sequences)
- Poorly-defined cervical and/or interosseous ligament
- Multiple cystic fluid collections hyperintense (FST2-FSE and STIR images)

Differential Diagnosis
Subtalar Arthrosis
- Subchondral sclerosis and chondral degeneration of middle and posterior facets

Pathology
General
- General Path Comments
  - Scarring and degenerative changes of soft-tissue structures
  - 70% history of inversion injury with lateral ligament complex tears
  - Tarsal canal contents include ligaments, posterior tibial and peroneal artery branches, veins, nerves and fat

Sinus Tarsi Syndrome

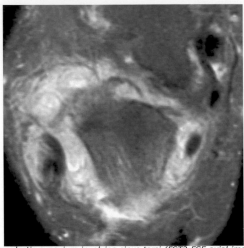

Hyperplastic synovium involving sinus tarsi (FST2-FSE axial image).

- o Tarsal canal ligaments
  - Inferior extensor retinaculum (medial, intermediate and lateral roots): Most superficial layer
  - Cervical ligament: Anterior (anterolateral) aspect of tarsal canal
  - Interosseous ligament: Medial (posteromedial) aspect of tarsal canal
- Etiology-Pathogenesis
  - o Trauma + subtalar microinstability

Clinical Issues
Presentation
- Heel instability, lateral ankle pain and tenderness over sinus tarsi
- 70% with history of inversion injury
- Association of posterior tibial tendon injury

Treatment & Prognosis
- Conservative; debridement

Selected References
1. Klein MA et al: MR imaging of the tarsal sinus and canal: Normal anatomy, pathologic findings, and features of the sinus tarsi syndrome. Radiology. 186:233, 1993
2. Lowe A et al: Sinus tarsi syndrome: A postoperative analysis. J Foot Surg. 24:108-12, 1985

Lisfranc Fracture - Dislocation

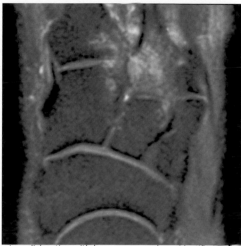

Lisfranc's fracture dislocation with bone marrow edema identified in first and second metatarsals proximally and medial cuneiform. There is lateral offset of the first metatarsal (FST2-FSE axial image).

Key Facts
- Homolateral: Lateral dislocation metatarsals
- Divergent (medial subluxation of first metatarsal and lateral dislocation metatarsals 2-5)
- Trauma and more commonly seen in neuropathic joint (diabetic charcot tarsometatarsal)

Imaging Findings
General Features
- Lateral offset proximal first metatarsal relative to medial cuneiform
- Lateral offset medial aspect second metatarsal relative to medial aspect intermediate cuneiform
- Associated fracture base second or third metatarsals, medial or intermediate cuneiform or navicular

MR Findings
- Marrow edema hyperintense on FST2-FSE or STIR images
- Dorsal displacement: Seen on direct coronal images

Differential Diagnosis
Bone Contusion Mid Foot
- Normal metatarsal cuneiform alignment without chip fracture or ligamentous disruption

Pathology
General
- Etiology-Pathogenesis
  - Forceful abduction of forefoot
  - Dislocations associated with fractures
  - No ligamentous connection between base of first and second metatarsals as normal anatomy

Lisfranc Fracture - Dislocation

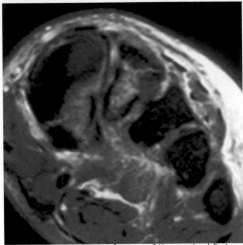

Corresponding coronal image showing fracture of the proximal first metatarsal and second metatarsal ((FST2-FSE coronal image).

Clinical Issues
Presentation
- Secondary to direct or indirect trauma

Treatment & Prognosis
- Anatomic reduction required

Selected References
1.   Vuori JP et al: Lisfranc joint injuries: Trauma mechanisms and associated injuries. J Trauma. 35:40, 1993
2.   Yamashita F et al: Diastasis between the medial and the intermediate cuneiforms. J Bone Joint Surg [Br]. 75:156, 1993
3.   Faciszewski T et al: Subtle injuries of the Lisfranc joint. J Bone Joint Surg [Am]. 72:1519, 1990

Os Trigonum Syndrome

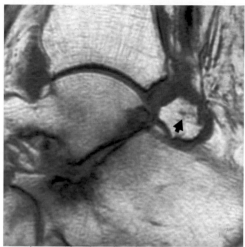

Os trigonum syndrome with enlarged os (arrow) and surrounding edema with tenosynovitis of the flexor hallucis longus tendon. Synchondrosis edema is present (T1-weighted sagittal images).

Key Facts
- Pathology of lateral tubercle posterior talar process
- Compression FHL tendon against medial edge of ununited lateral tubercle
- Includes posterior ankle impingement and talar compression syndrome
- Pain with disruption of cartilaginous synchondrosis between os trigonum and lateral tubercle talus

Imaging Findings
MR Findings
- Hyperintense synovitis posterior to os trigonum (FST2-FSE or STIR)
- Hyperintense os trigonum on T2 (FST2-FSE)
- Isolated tenosynovitis flexor hallucis longus (FHL) tendon sheath (partial tethering of FHL tendon): May not have associated tibiotalar joint effusion
- Degenerative cystic changes between os trigonum and talus

Differential Diagnosis
Chronic Ununited Fracture of Lateral Tubercle
- Os trigonum represents congenital nonunion of lateral tubercle of posterior talar process

Pathology
General
- Etiology-Pathogenesis
  - Repetitive microtrauma and chronic inflammation with soft-tissue thickening
  - Other etiologies: Trigonal process fracture, FHL tenosynovitis, posterior tibiotalar bony impingement and intraarticular loose bodies

Os Trigonum Syndrome

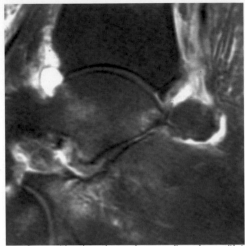

Os trigonum syndrome with enlarged os and surrounding edema with tenosynovitis of the flexor hallucis longus tendon. Synchondrosis edema is present (FST2-FSE sagittal image).

- ○ Ununited lateral tubercle (50% bilateral)
- ○ Presence of os trigonum not required for diagnosis

Clinical Issues

Presentation

- Chronic pain, stiffness, tenderness, soft-tissue swelling in posterior ankle
- Extreme plantar flexion with compression and entrapment of synovial capsular tissue against posterior tibia
- Associated FHL tenosynovitis

Treatment & Prognosis

- Conservative versus surgical excision

Selected References
1. Karasick D et al: The os trigonum syndrome: Imaging features. AJR. 166:125, 1996
2. Marotta JJ et al: Os trigonum impingement in dancers. Am J Sports Med. 20:23, 1992

Plantaris Rupture

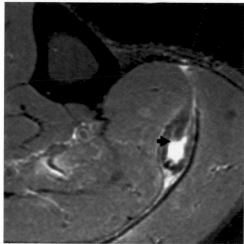

Plantaris tendon rupture (arrow) with a mass of tissue and intermuscular hemorrhage between soleus and medial head of the gastrocnemius muscle groups (FST2-FSE axial image).

Key Facts
- Myotendinous junction rupture
- Acute calf pain + swelling and ecchymosis
- Knee extension with ankle dorsiflexion

Imaging Findings
MR Findings
- Intermuscular hematoma: Between medial head gastrocnemius and soleus
- Retracted plantaris tendon + hemorrhage with mass of intermediate signal intensity blood and tissue
- Hypointense signal in area of hemorrhage secondary to susceptibility on T2*-weighted images
- Associated muscle strain of medial head gastrocnemius with hyperintense interstitial signal intensity on FST2-FSE or STIR images
- Hyperintense fluid in plane of hematoma extends medially toward deep subcutaneous tissue
- Proximal muscle strain at level of knee joint associated with ACL and posterolateral corner injuries
- Proximal ruptures: Retracted tendon between popliteus tendon and lateral head gastrocnemius

Differential Diagnosis
Strain of the Medial Head of the Gastrocnemius and Soleus
- Includes injuries of the musculotendinous unit (MTU)
- Normal course of plantaris tendon from lateral proximally to medially distally

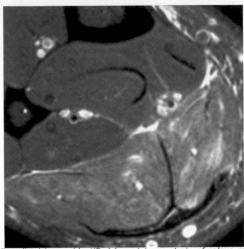

Corresponding distal image identified hyperintense strain of soleus muscle group (FST2-FSE axial image).

Pathology
<u>General</u>
- General Path Comments
  - o Isolated or associated with partial tear of the gastrocnemius or popliteus muscle
  - o Myotendinous junction of plantaris at level of soleus origin on tibia
- Etiology-Pathogenesis
  - o Acute injury with hematoma

Clinical Issues
<u>Presentation</u>
- Impaired gait locomotion and toe off portion of stance phase
- Calf hemorrhage associated with aching and cramping pain
- Palpable knot or deficit on clinical exam
- Tennis leg = proximal tendon rupture

<u>Treatment & Prognosis</u>
- Conservative treatment
- Complication: Posterior compartment syndrome

Selected References
1. Helms CA et al: Plantaris muscle injury: Evaluation with MR imaging. Radiology. 195:201, 1995
2. Anouchi YS et al: Posterior compartment syndrome of the calf resulting from misdiagnosis of a rupture of the medial head of the gastrocnemius. J Trauma. 27:678, 1987
3. Froimson AE: Tennis leg. JAMA. 209:415, 1969

Tarsal Tunnel

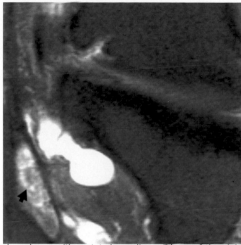

Tarsal tunnel syndrome with septated ganglion. Edema of the abductor hallucis (arrow) is shown medially (FST2-FSE coronal image).

Key Facts
- Entrapment or compression neuropathy of posterior tibial nerve in fibro-osseous tunnel deep to flexor retinaculum
- Posteroinferior to medial malleolus
- Pain + sensory deficits sole of foot and intrinsic muscle weakness

Imaging Findings
MR Findings
- Hyperintense signal from ganglion cyst (FST2-FSE and STIR) from FHL tendon sheath (septated and multiloculated)
- Fibrosis: Hypointense on T1 and T2 (FST2-FSE and STIR)
- Varicose veins: Serpiginous vascular hyperintense signal on T2
- IV contrast to enhance neural tumors (T2* contrast also useful in neural tumor histology)
- IV contrast enhances synovial hypertrophy

Differential Diagnosis
Anterior Tarsal Tunnel Syndrome
- Compression of deep peroneal nerve beneath inferior extensor retinaculum
Distal Entrapment
- Talonavicular or naviculocuneiform osteophytes

Pathology
General
- Etiology-Pathogenesis
  - Tarsal tunnel posterior and inferior to medial malleolus
  - Posterior tibial nerve trifurcates into medial and lateral plantar nerves + sensory calcaneal branches distal to medial malleolus

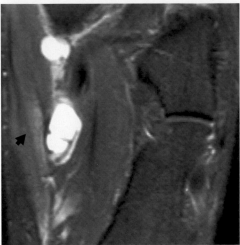

Corresponding axial image with hyperintense ganglion and edema of the abductor hallucis (arrow) are shown (FST2-FSE axial image).

- ○ Compression neuropathy: Lipomas, varicose veins (common finding), ganglion, neurilemmomas, scarring, tenosynovitis and accessory muscles
- ○ Entrapment posterior tibial nerve

Gross Pathologic or Surgical Features
- • Surgical findings: Entrapment of flexor retinaculum; fibrous origin abductor hallucis muscle; tenosynovitis; post-traumatic fibrosis

Clinical Issues
Presentation
- • Pain, paresthesias + motor dysfunction in distribution of posterior tibial nerve

Treatment & Prognosis
- • Conservative or surgical decompression (increased success if specific lesion identified within tarsal tunnel)

Selected References
1. Pfeiffer WH et al: Clinical results after tarsal tunnel decompression. J Bone Joint Surg [Am]. 76A: 1222, 1994
2. Zeiss J et al: Normal magnetic resonance anatomy of the tarsal tunnel. Foot Ankle. 10:214, 1990
3. Erickson SJ et al: MR imaging of the tarsal tunnel and related spaces: Normal and abnormal findings with anatomic correlation. AJR. 155:323, 1990

Morton's Neuroma

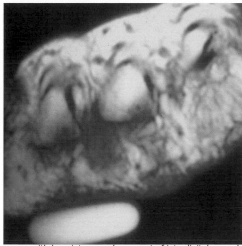

Morton's neuroma with hypointense enlargement of the interdigital nerve between third and fourth metatarsal heads (T1-weighted coronal image).

Key Facts
- Metatarsalgia with localized enlargement of the interdigital nerve between the third and fourth metatarsal heads
- Lateral branch medial plantar nerve to third interspace
- Women 40 to 60 years of age

Imaging Findings
MR Findings
- Hypointense on T1-weighted coronal images
- Intermediate to increased signal intensity on fat suppressed T2FSE and STIR images
- T2*: Intermediate to increased signal intensity
- Area of involvement between plantar aspects of involved metatarsal heads
- Epineurium fibrosis intermediate signal on T1 and (FST2-FSE)
- Contrast enhanced MR most sensitive

Differential Diagnosis
Neurofibroma
- Hyperintense on conventional T2 and FST2-FSE images
- Morton's neuroma requires STIR or FST2-FSE to show intermediate to increased signal intensity (hypointense on conventional T2-weighted images)

Pathology
General
- Etiology-Pathogenesis
    - Metatarsalgia with localized enlargement of the interdigital nerve between the third and fourth metatarsal heads
    - Fibrotic response: Not true tumor

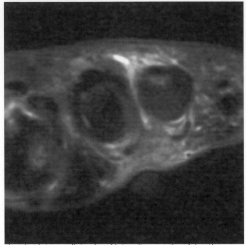

STIR image showing intermediate signal intensity mass involving the second interspace on the plantar aspect of the foot (STIR coronal image in a separate case).

<u>Microscopic Features</u>
- Deposition of eosinophilic material
- Degeneration of nerve fibers secondary to entrapment neuropathy

Clinical Issues
<u>Presentation</u>
- Plantar foot pain
- Tenderness of the involved interspace
- Women 40 to 60 years of age

<u>Treatment & Prognosis</u>
- Surgical excision

Selected References
1. Terk MR et al: Morton neuroma: Evaluation with MR imaging performed with contrast enhancement and fat suppression. Radiology. 189:239, 1993
2. Satoris DJ et al: Magnetic resonance images. Interdigital or Morton's neuroma. J Foot Surg. 28:78, 1989

AVN of the Talus

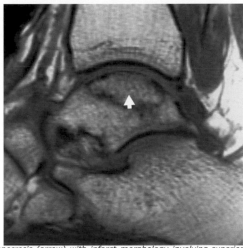

Talar osteonecrosis (arrow) with infarct morphology involving superior talar dome (T1-weighted sagittal image).

Key Facts
- AVN (avascular necrosis): Body of the talus
- Associated with talar neck fractures
- +/- subtalar dislocation
- Two MR patterns: Localized ischemia + diffuse bone marrow edema versus diffuse infarction pattern

Imaging Findings
MR Findings
- Initially small, hypointense focus of necrosis superior talar dome + disproportionate diffuse marrow edema hyperintense on T2-weighted images (FST2FSE or STIR)
- Marrow edema is most intense adjacent ischemic focus (edema hypointense T1, hyperintense T2)
- Chronic appearance: Resolution of bone marrow edema with persistent, well-demarcated focus of osteonecrosis (edema is never seen without focus of AVN)
- Diffuse talar osteonecrosis: Bone infarct morphology

Differential Diagnosis
OCL
- Less extensive marrow edema in early stages
Infection
- Erosion, without sclerotic focus
Tumor
- No superior talar necrotic focus

Pathology
General
- Etiology-Pathogenesis
  - Associated with talar neck fractures

AVN of the Talus

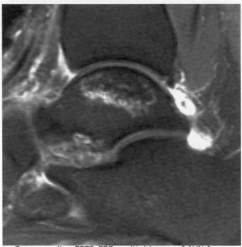

Corresponding FST2-FSE sagittal image of AVN focus.

- +/- subtalar dislocation
- Blood supply from tarsal canal artery, a posterior tibial artery branch
- Talar injuries + subtalar joint disruption – 40-50% rate of AVN
- +/- collapse of articular cartilage

Clinical Issues
<u>Presentation</u>
- Acute ankle pain (decreases with resolution of marrow edema)
- Bilateral involvement with asynchrony not uncommon

<u>Treatment & Prognosis</u>
- Decreased weightbearing and possible decompression for pain with marrow edema

Selected References:
1. Mitchell MJ: The foot and ankle. Top Magn Reson Imaging. 1:57-73, 1989
2. Hawkins LG: Fractures of the neck of the talus J Bone Joint Surg Am. 52A: 991-1002, 1970

Plantar Fasciitis

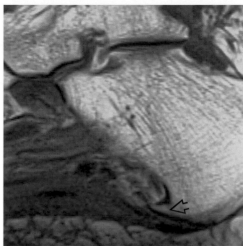

Plantar fasciitis with fat marrow (arrow) containing enthesophyte (T1-weighted sagittal image).

Key Facts
- Inflammation of plantar aponeurosis
- Associated calcaneal spur, inflammatory changes and/or thickening
- Hyperintensity of plantar aponeurosis adjacent to os calcis attachment

Imaging Findings
MR Findings
- Hyperintensity in thickened (7 to 8 mm) plantar fascial attachment to the os calcis +/- enthesophyte
- Hyperintense edema of the soft tissues (perifascial structures) plantar to os calcis attachment of plantar aponeurosis
- Partial detachment of medial or lateral cord
- Coronal MR images define lateral and medial cord versus central attachment
- Sagittal MR images define long axis of plantar fascia

Differential Diagnosis
Plantar Fibromatosis
- Hypointense nodules on T1, intermediate to increased signal intensity on FST2-FSE or STIR images
- Distal to os calcis attachment

Pathology
General
- General Path Comments
  - Subcalcaneal pain syndrome: Microtrauma of plantar fascia with attempted repair and chronic inflammation
  - Plantar fascia aggravated by pes planus and hyperpronation
  - +/- Nerve entrapment or irritation of the medial calcaneal nerve or lateral plantar branch to abductor digiti quinti

Plantar Fasciitis

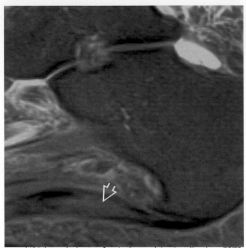

Hyperintense and thickened plantar fascia (arrow) is visualized on FST2-FSE sagittal image.

- Etiology-Pathogenesis
  - Mechanical: (Pes cavus) pronated foot
  - Degenerative: Increased foot pronation, calcaneal heel pad atrophy
  - Systemic: Rheumatoid arthritis and seronegative spondyloarthropathies

Microscopic Features
- Angiofibroblastic hyperplasia
- Collagen degeneration
- Calcification

Clinical Issues

Presentation
- Pain medial tuberosity calcaneus (pain with dorsiflexion of the toes)
- Plantar calcaneal enthesophyte (50%)

Treatment & Prognosis
- Initial treatment conservative with stretching of plantar fascia prior to surgical division

Selected References
1. Narvaez JA et al: Painful heel: MR image findings. Radiographics. 20:333-52, 2000
2. Grasel RP et al: MR imaging of plantar fasciitis edema, tears and occult marrow abnormalities correlated with outcome. AJR.173: 699-701, 1999

BONE MARROW

Langerhans Cell Histiocytosis

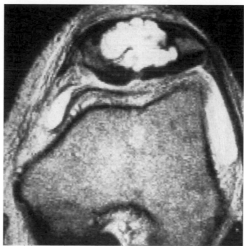

Lesion of eosinophilic granuloma with complication of pathologic fracture in the patella (T2-weighted axial image).

Key Facts
- Represents <1% of all biopsy-proven primary bone lesions
- Incidence: 0.05-0.5 per 100 000 children per year in the US

Imaging Findings
General Features
- Calvarium > mandible > long bones (meta-/diaphysis) > ribs > pelvis > vertebrae
- Monostotic involvement: 50-75%
- Multifocal involvement: 10-20%
MR Findings
- T1 MR: Low SI
- T2 MR: High SI
Plain Film Findings
- Skull (50%)
  - Well-defined lytic lesion without sclerotic rim
  - Sclerotic rim during healing phase
  - Occasional cortical destruction
  - Coalescence of lesions, geographic skull
  - Hole-within-a-hole appearance: Outer table of skull more destroyed than inner table; button sequestrum
  - Soft-tissue mass overlying lytic process in calvarium
  - Floating tooth: Lesion in alveolar portion of mandible
- Appendicular skeleton
  - Expansile lytic lesion with ill-defined/sclerotic edges
  - Endosteal scalloping, widening of medullary cavity
  - Lesions respect joint space/growth plate
- Spine and pelvis (25%)
  - Vertebra plana: Complete collapse of vertebral body

Langerhans Cell Histiocytosis

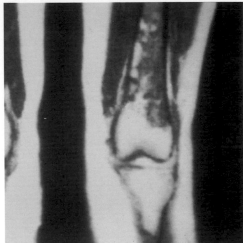

Eosinophilic granuloma (of histiocytosis X) affecting the femoral diaphysis and metaphysis with patchy, hypointense areas of histiocytic infiltration (T1-weighted coronal image).

Differential Diagnosis

Osteomyelitis
- Moth-eaten appearance
- Periosteal reaction

Ewing's Sarcoma
- Permeative bone destruction
- Lamellated periosteal reaction
- Progression of tumor (DD Langerhans histiocytosis: "Tempo phenomenon" rapid progression and disappearance of lesion)

Pathology

General
- Etiology-Pathogenesis
  - Group of disorders involving abnormal proliferation of histiocytes in organs of RES
    - Letterer-Siwe: Acute disseminated form, 10%
    - Hand Schueller Christian: Chronic disseminated form: 20%
    - Eosinophilic granuloma: Only bone involvement, 70%

Gross Pathologic or Surgical Features
- Yellow, gray, or brown tumor mass with hemorrhagic areas

Microscopic Features
- Proliferation of Langerhans cells (produce prostaglandin -> causes bone resorption)
- Infiltrate of histiocytes, eosinophils, lymphocytes, neutrophils, plasma cells

Clinical Issues

Presentation
- Age: 2-30 years, mean age: 5-10 years, M:F=2:1
- Local pain, tenderness
- Swelling/ soft-tissue mass

Langerhans Cell Histiocytosis

- Fever, elevated sedimentation rate, leukocytosis

Treatment & Prognosis
- Observation
- Excision and curettage
- Radiation therapy
- Eosinophilic granuloma has best prognosis with spontaneous remission of bone lesions

Selected References
1. Lieberman PH et al: Langerhans cell (eosinophilic) granulomatosis. A clinicopathologic study encompassing 50 years. Am J Surg Pathol. 20:519-52, 1996
2. Fisher AJ et al: Quantitative analysis of the plain radiographic appearance of eosinophilic granuloma. Invest Radiol. 30:466-73, 1995
3. Beltran J et al: Eosinophilic granuloma: MRI manifestations. Skeletal Radiol. 22:157-61, 1993

Leukemia

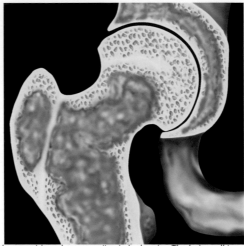

Marrow replacement in red marrow sites in leukemia. The hairy cell type of leukemia has a more nodular or patchy pattern of marrow replacement.

Key Facts
- Most common malignancy of childhood
- Represents 20th most common cause of cancer death in all age groups

Imaging Findings
General Features
- Children: Long bones
- Adults: Axial skeleton

Plain Film Findings
- Diffuse osteopenia of spine and long bones
  - ○ Coarse trabeculation of spongiosa
  - ○ Multiple partially collapsed vertebrae
- "Leukemic lines" (40-53% in ALL)
  - ○ Transverse, radiolucent metaphyseal bands involving large joints
  - ○ Horizontal bands in vertebral bodies
  - ○ Dense metaphyseal lines post therapy
- Focal destruction of flat/ tubular bones
  - ○ Multiple small clearly-defined osteolytic lesions
  - ○ Moth eaten appearance
  - ○ Sutural widening, prominent convolutional markings of skull
- Periostitis of long bones
  - ○ Smooth/ lamellated/ sunburst pattern of periosteal reaction (12-25%)

MR Findings
- T1 MR: Low SI (leukemic infiltrate) replacing high SI marrow fat
- T2 MR: Increased SI
- STIR: Increased SI of leukemic marrow

Leukemia

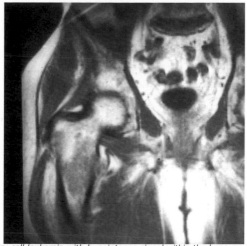

Hairy cell leukemia with hypointense signal within the bone marrow.

Differential Diagnosis
Metastatic Neuroblastoma
- Bone involvement similar to leukemia: metaphyseal bands, moth eaten bone destruction
- Hair-on-end appearance of skull

Langerhans Cell Histiocytosis
- Lytic lesion with sclerotic margin
- Periosteal reaction
- Soft-tissue mass

Pathology
General
- General Path Comments
  - Classified as acute/ chronic lymphocytic or myelogenous form
  - Clinical and radiographic signs of bone marrow involvement typically in children with acute leukemia
- Etiology-Pathogenesis
  - Arises from primitive stem cell either de novo or from preexisting preleukemic state

Gross Pathologic or Surgical Features
- Hyperemic/ hemorrhagic bone marrow with destruction of bony trabeculae or osteosclerosis
- Areas of bone infarction

Microscopic Features
- Typical childhood form ALL: Patternless sheets of small blue cells
- Infiltration of bone marrow by poorly-differentiated blast cells

Clinical Issues
Presentation
- Sharp, localized, recurrent paraarticular arthralgias (in 75%)

Leukemia

- Joint effusion
- Fever, elevated ESR
- May be confused with acute rheumatic fever, rheumatoid arthritis, osteomyelitis
- Hepatosplenomegaly

Treatment & Prognosis
- Chemotherapy
- Bone marrow transplant

Selected References
1. Gallagher DJ et al: Orthopedic manifestations of acute pediatric leukemia. Orthop Clin North Am. 27:635-44, 1996
2. Heinrich SD et al: The prognostic significance of the skeletal manifestations of acute lymphoblastic leukemia of childhood. J Pediatr Orthop. 14:105-11, 1994
3. Oestreich AE: Imaging of the skeleton and soft tissues in children. Curr Opin Radiol. 4:55-61, 1992

Lymphoma

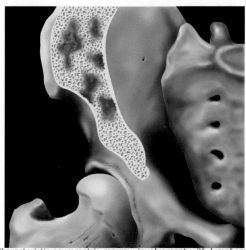

Characteristic asymmetric marrow involvement with lymphoma.

Key Facts
- Primary osseous lymphoma represents 3%-4% of all malignant bone tumors
- Skeletal system may be secondary involved in 30% of malignant lymphomas

Imaging Findings
General Features
- Dia-metaphysis of lower femur, upper tibia (40% around the knee)
- Humerus, pelvis, scapulae, ribs, vertebrae

Plain Film Findings
- Cancellous bone erosion (earliest sign)
- Mottled permeative pattern of separate coalescent areas
- Edges of lesion blend imperceptibly with normal bone (plain film often grossly underestimates extent of tumor)
- Late cortical destruction with associated soft-tissue mass
- "Ivory bone" in vertebrae or flat bones

CT Findings
- To determine bone destruction and soft-tissue involvement
- Can detect bony sequestrum (occur in 11%)

MR Findings
- T1 MR: Diffuse infiltration low SI
- T2 MR: Involved areas hyperintense to muscle
- STIR: Lymphomatous infiltration high SI

Bone Scan Findings
- Increased uptake
- Combination of normal plain radiographs and positive bone scan should suggest possibility of osseous lymphoma

Differential Diagnosis
Ewing Sarcoma
- Systemic symptoms

Lymphoma

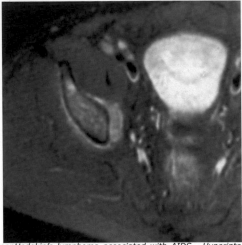

Large cell nonHodgkin's lymphoma associated with AIDS. Hyperintense marrow involves right iliac bone marrow (FST2-FSE axial image).

- Younger patients
- Lamellated/onion skin periosteal reaction

Chronic Osteomyelitis
- Can have similar radiographic picture
- Systemic symptoms

Osteosarcoma
- Less medullary extension
- Younger patients

Pathology
General
- Etiology-Pathogenesis
  - Primary osseous lymphoma: Arises within medullary cavity of single bone without concurrent lymph node or visceral involvement for at least six months following diagnosis
  - Majority of cases are of non-Hodgkin type (large cell type)

Gross Pathologic or Surgical Features
- Soft, fleshy, intraosseous component (centered in metaphyses) with mixture of bone spicules and marrow fat and areas of necrosis
- Indistinct margins
- Extraosseous tissue with tan/ white appearance, resembles lymphomatous lymph nodes

Microscopic Features
- Aggregates of malignant, small, round, lymphocytic cells that fill marrow spaces
- Hodgkin's lymphoma: Reed-Sternberg cells

Clinical Issues
Presentation
- Age: 20-70 years, peak age: 35-45 years, M:F=1.5-2:1
- Localized dull/aching pain

Lymphoma

- 50% of patients have symptoms for over one year
- Occasionally palpable mass
- Pathologic fractures in 25%

<u>Treatment & Prognosis</u>
- Radiation and chemotherapy
- Surgery in cases of pathologic fractures
- Primary osseous lymphoma without soft tissue involvement has best prognosis of all osseous malignancies

Selected References
1. Jones D et al: Lymphoma presenting as a solitary bone lesion. Am J Clin Pathol. 111:171-8, 1999
2. Hillemanns M et al: Malignant lymphoma. Skeletal Radiol. 25:73-5, 1996
3. Bragg DG: Radiology of the lymphomas. Curr Probl Diagn Radiol. 16:177-206, 1987

Sickle Cell Anemia

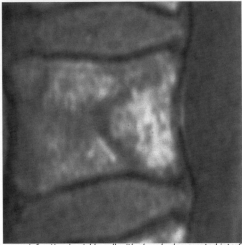

Vertebral marrow infarction in sickle cell with sharply demarcated interface between normal marrow and ischemic marrow (T1-weighted sagittal image).

Key Facts
- Affects 1% of African Americans
- 8-13% of African Americans carry sickling factor (HbS)

Imaging Findings
MR Findings
- T1 MR: Diffusely low SI of bone marrow (hematopoietic marrow replacing fatty marrow)
- T2 MR: Diffusely low SI of bone marrow (hematopoietic marrow replacing fatty marrow)
  - Focal areas of increased SI (acute marrow infarction)

Plain Film Findings
- Biconcave H-vertebra (bone softening) (70%)
- Osteoporosis with thinning of trabeculae
- Hair-on-end appearance of skull (vertical striations)
- Widening of medullary space, thinning of cortex
- AVN in medullary spaces of long bones, hands, growing epiphyses
  - Periosteal reaction: Bone-within-bone appearance
  - Bone sclerosis from infarction
  - Collapse of femoral head
  - Dactylitis (hand-foot syndrome): Bone infarcts of hands and feet

Bone Scan Findings
- Symmetric, marked expansion of hematopoietic marrow involving femur, calvarium, small bones of hand and feet
- Bone marrow defects (acute/ old disease)

Differential Diagnosis
Thalassemia
- Expanded bone marrow space
- H-shaped vertebra
- Hair-on-end skull

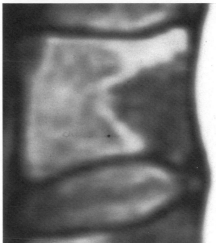

Corresponding hyperintense marrow of infarction in sickle cell anemia (T2-FSE sagittal image).

- AVN less common than in sickle cell anemia
- Paravertebral masses (extramedullary hematopoiesis)

Pathology
General
- Etiology-Pathogenesis
  - Structural defect in hemoglobin Hb S: Glutamic acid in position 6 substituted with Valin
  - Sickle cell disease (HbSS) associated with many bone findings, sickle cell trait (HbAS) occasionally associated with bone infarcts

Gross Pathologic or Surgical Features
- Yellow necrotic subchondral bone separated from overlying articular cartilage and surrounded by a rim of fibrous tissue and sclerotic bone trabeculae
- Produces crescent-shaped defect (characteristic radiographic "crescent sign")

Microscopic Features
- Altered shape and plasticity of RBCs under lowered oxygen tension lead to increased blood viscosity, stasis
- Occlusion of small blood vessels lead to infarction

Clinical Issues
Presentation
- Crises begin at 2-3 years of age and may lead to bone infarctions
- Skeletal pain (bone marrow infarction, osteomyelitis, cellulitis)
- Osteomyelitis: In diaphysis of long bones (Salmonella, Staphylococcus)
- Hemolytic anemia, jaundice
- Abdominal pain
- Splenomegaly (in children), later splenic atrophy
- High incidence of infections
- Chest pain: Acute pulmonary crisis, infarcts

Sickle Cell Anemia

<u>Treatment & Prognosis</u>
- Sickle cell crisis: Oxygen, hydration, pain management
- High-dose methylprednisolone can reduce duration of pain in children
- Death < 40 years in sickle cell disease

Selected References
1. Jean-Baptiste G et al: Osteoarticular disorders of haematological origin. Baillieres Best Pract Res Clin Rheumatol. 14:307-23, 2000
2. Rao VM et al: Femoral head avascular necrosis in sickle cell anemia: MR characteristics. Magn Reson Imaging. 6:661-7, 1988

Metastases

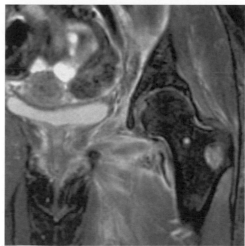

Metastatic lung carcinoma post radiation of left hemipelvis. Tumor is present in left greater trochanter (FST2-FSE coronal image).

Key Facts
- Bone marrow is the third most common site of metastatic disease
- Metastases to bone 25 times more common than primary skeletal neoplasms

Imaging Findings
General Features
- Axial skeleton more frequently involved than appendicular skeleton (persistence of red marrow in axial skeleton)
- Ribs, pelvis, spine, skull, femur, humerus most common sites
- Distal bones rarely affected
- Metastases can be osteoblastic, lytic, or mixed
- Single/multiple lesions of variable size
- Joint spaces and intervertebral spaces preserved (cartilage resistant to invasion)

MR Findings
- Lytic metastases
  - T1 MR: Low SI
  - T2 MR: High SI
- Osteoblastic metastases
  - T1 MR: Low SI
  - T2 MR: Low SI
- Mixed metastases
  - T1 MR: Inhomogeneously low SI
  - T2 MR: Inhomogeneously high SI

Bone Scan Findings
- High sensitivity for many metastatic tumors (breast, lung, prostate)
- 5% of bone marrow metastases have normal bone scan
- Multiple asymmetric areas of increased uptake
- Superscan in diffuse bone marrow metastases
- Decreased activity in osteolytic metastases

Metastases

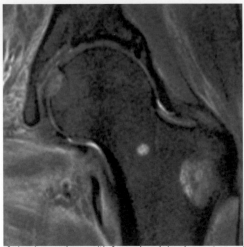

Small field of view image shown with femoral neck involvement as well as greater trochanter. Radiation myositis produces adductor muscle hyperintensity (FST2-FSE coronal image).

Differential Diagnosis
Multiple Myeloma
- Late involvement of pedicles (pedicles involved first in metastases)
- Cold on bone scan

Pathology
General
- Etiology-Pathogenesis
  - Hematogenous spread through arterial circulation to vascular red marrow
  - Hematogenous spread through retrograde venous flow (e.g. prostate)
  - Direct extension (uncommon)
  - Cancers most likely to metastasize to bone include breast, lung, prostate, thyroid, kidney
    - Children: neuroblastoma
Gross Pathologic or Surgical Features
- Firm, whitish tumor with or without necrotic, hemorrhagic areas (especially in renal cell cancer)
Microscopic Features
- Replacement of bone marrow by carcinoma cells depending on the origin of the primary tumor
- Excretion of osteoclast-stimulating factors by metastatic cells

Clinical Issues
Presentation
- Pain (70%), pathologic fractures, hypercalcemia (10%)
- Neurologic impairment in spinal metastases

Metastases

Treatment & Prognosis
- Osteoclast inhibiting agents: Bisphosphates
- Radiation therapy
- Patients with lung cancers and bone marrow metastases: Median survival is less than six months

Selected References
1. Vanel D et al: MRI of bone marrow disorders. Eur Radiol. 10:224-9, 2000
2. Traill ZC et al: Magnetic resonance imaging versus radionuclide scintigraphy in screening for bone metastases. Clin Radiol. 54:448-51, 1999
3. Vanel D et al: MRI of bone metastases. Eur Radiol. 8:1345-51, 1998

Multiple Myeloma

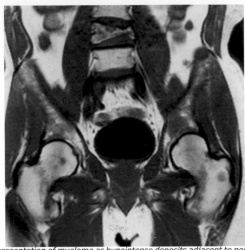

Multifocal presentation of myeloma as hypointense deposits adjacent to normal marrow (T1-weighted coronal image).

Key Facts
- Most common primary tumor of bone
- Accounts for 27% of biopsied bone tumors

Imaging Findings
General Features
- Involvement of bones that contain red marrow: Axial skeleton (spine, skull (mandible), ribs, pelvis) > long bones
- Plain film
  - Multiple, well-circumscribed, punched-out lesions (80%)
  - Endosteal scalloping
  - Soft-tissue mass adjacent to bone destruction
  - Diffuse osteoporosis or osteolysis
  - Expansile osteolytic lesion (ribs, pelvis, long bones)
- Plasmocytoma: Solitary, large, expansile lesion (ribs, pelvis)
  - Represents early stage of multiple myeloma
- POEMS syndrome: Polyneuropathy, organomegaly, endocrine disorders, monoclonal gammopathy, skin changes
  - Enthesopathies of posterior elements of thoracic and lumbar spine
  - Lytic lesions with surrounding sclerosis

MR Findings
- T1 MR: Intermediate SI compared to surrounding bone
- T2 MR: Homogeneous high SI

Bone Scan Findings
- Normal scan in majority of cases
- Detects 10% of lesions

Differential Diagnosis
Metastases
- Pedicles involved first (late involvement in myeloma)
- Increased activity on bone scan

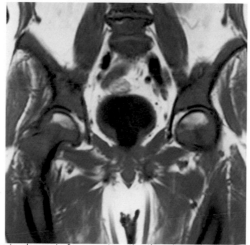

Diffuse involvement of marrow targeting the spine and pelvis in multiple myeloma.

- Usually does **not** involve mandible

Severe Osteoporosis
- No endosteal scalloping

Pathology
General
- Etiology-Pathogenesis
  - ○ Characterized by uncontrolled proliferation of plasma cells within bone marrow that secrete nonfunctional monoclonal immunoglobulins

Gross Pathologic or Surgical Features
- Confluent or well-circumscribed, red-gray, soft tumor replacing cancellous bone

Microscopic Features
- Aggregates neoplastic plasma cells infiltrate and completely replace normal hematopoietic and fatty marrow
- The myeloma cells: Eccentric, round, hyperchromatic nucleus with "cartwheel" distribution of chromatin

Clinical Issues
Presentation
- Age: 40-80 years, peak age: 64 years, M:F=3:2
- Mild transient bone pain, worsened by activity (75%)
- Anemia, fever, weight loss
- Hypercalcemia
- Bence Jones proteins in urine
- Electrophoresis: Monoclonal gammopathy (IgA/ IgG peak)
- Pathologic fractures
- Amyloidosis (10%)

Multiple Myeloma

Treatment & Prognosis
- Radiation and chemotherapy
- Osteoclast inhibiting agents: Bisphosphates
- Survival time 3 to 5 years with chemotherapy

Selected References
1. Lecouvet FE et al: Skeletal survey in advanced multiple myeloma: Radiographic versus MR imaging survey. Br J Haematol. 106:35-9, 1999
2. Libshitz HI et al: Multiple myeloma: Appearance at MR imaging. Radiology. 182:833-7, 1992
3. Moulopoulos LA et al: Multiple myeloma: Spinal MR imaging in patients with untreated newly diagnosed disease. Radiology. 185:833-40, 1992

Gaucher's Disease

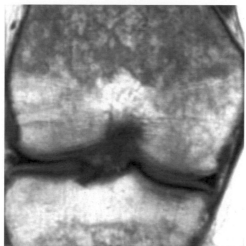

Gaucher's disease with hypointense signal from lipid in reticuloendothelial cells (T1-weighted coronal image).

Key Facts
- Rare autosomal recessive disorder which is common among Ashkenazi Jewish population
- Most common genetic lysosomal storage disorder

Imaging Findings
General Features
- Involves the axial skeleton, distal femur, pelvis, other long bones

Plain Film Findings
- Generalized osteopenia
- Erosion of inner cortex and widened medullary cavity
- Endosteal scalloping
- Multiple well-circumscribed lytic lesions
- Erlenmeyer flask deformity of distal femur, proximal tibia
- Weakened subchondral bone, degenerative arthritis
- H-shaped vertebrae
- Osteonecrosis

MR Findings
- T1 MR: Patchy, coarse areas of decreased SI
- T2 MR: Decreased SI
- STIR MR: Increased SI

Differential Diagnosis
Multiple Myeloma
- Older age group
- Soft-tissue mass adjacent to bone destruction

Mucopolysaccharidoses
- Shortened extremity bones
- Short, thick finger bones
- Hypoplastic pelvis

Gaucher's Disease

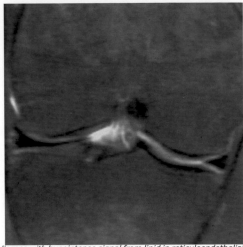

Gaucher's disease with hypointense signal from lipid in reticuloendothelial cells (FST2-FSE coronal image).

Pathology
General
- Etiology-Pathogenesis
  - Deficiency of beta-glucocerebrosidase leads to accumulation of glucosylceramide within cells of RES
  - Gene for glucocerebrosidase located on chromosome 1q21

Gross Pathologic or Surgical Features
- Infiltration of cancellous bone with pale yellow tissue distinguishable from fatty marrow

Microscopic Features
- Infiltration of bone marrow with Gaucher cells (kerasin-laden histiocytes)
- Gaucher cell: Large, pale, polyhedral-shaped cell with single eccentric nucleus and weakly eosinophilic cytoplasm containing striations ("wrinkled tissue paper" appearance)

Clinical Issues
Presentation
- Adult (type I), infantile (type II), and juvenile (type III)
- M<F
- Hepatosplenomegaly
- Pancytopenia (hypersplenism)
- Pathologic fractures
- Osteomyelitis
- Repeated pulmonary infections
- Osteoarthritis

Gaucher's Disease

<u>Treatment & Prognosis</u>
- Beta-glucosidase mannose substitution
  - ○ Substitution of mannose to the enzyme glucosidase causes destruction of the accumulated glucosylceramide
- AVN: Bed rest and analgesics, total hip replacement in advanced cases
- Adult form (type I): Longest time of survival

Selected References
1. Hermann G et al: Assessment of skeletal involvement and therapeutic responses to enzyme replacement. Skeletal Radiol. 26:687-97, 1997
2. Oestreich AE: Imaging of the skeleton and soft tissues in children. Curr Opin Radiol. 4:55-61, 1992

Paget's Disease

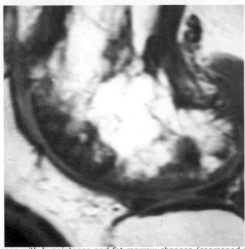

Paget's disease with hypointense and fat marrow changes (coarsened appearance) in distal femur (T1-weighted sagittal image).

Key Facts
- Affects 3% of individuals over 40 years and 10% of over 80 years

Imaging Findings
General Features
- Pelvis, 75% > spine > femur > skull > tibia > clavicle > humerus > ribs
- Polyostotic, asymmetric
- Long bones: Lesion starts at one end of bone, extend along shaft

Plain Film Findings
- Pelvis
  - Thickening of iliopectineal line
  - Thickened trabeculae, coarse cortex
  - Acetabular protrusion
- Skull
  - Diploic widening: Inner and outer table involved
  - Osteoporosis circumscripta: Well-defined lysis (destructive active stage)
  - Cotton-wool appearance: Mixed lytic and blastic pattern of thickened calvarium (late stage)
  - Basilar invagination with narrowing of foramen magnum
- Long bones
  - "Candle flame" lysis: V-shaped lytic defect originating in subarticular site advancing into diaphysis of long bone
  - Banana fractures: Small, horizontal stress fractures (lateral bowing of femur, anterior bowing of tibia)
- Spine
  - Picture-frame vertebral body: Enlarged, square, vertebral body with thickened, peripheral trabeculae and radiolucent inner portion
  - Ivory vertebra: Increased density

MR Findings
- T1 MR: Low SI, coarsened appearance of bone marrow

Paget's Disease

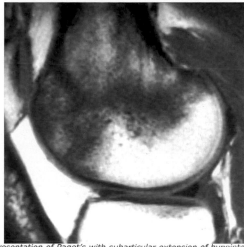

Sclerotic presentation of Paget's with subarticular extension of hypointense marrow changes (T1-weighted sagittal image).

- T2 MR: Low SI

CT Findings
- Dense enhancement in lytic phase
- Bone scan
- Useful in determining extent of disease
- Increased uptake in lytic phase
- Normal scan in sclerotic, burned-out lesions

Differential Diagnosis
Osteoblastic Metastases
- May be indistinguishable

Lymphoma
- Cancellous bone erosion
- Cortical destruction with soft-tissue mass
- T2 MR: High SI of involved areas

Fibrous Dysplasia
- Ground glass appearance
- Cranial lesions may be indistinguishable

Pathology
General
- Etiology-Pathogenesis
  o Chronic disease of osteoblasts and osteoclasts resulting in abnormal bone remodeling
  o Possible viral etiology
  o Sarcomatous transformation (< 1%): into osteosarcoma (22-90%), fibrosarcoma/MFH (29-51%), chondrosarcoma (1-15%)

Gross Pathologic or Surgical Features
- Newly formed bone abnormally soft and deformed

Paget's Disease

Microscopic Features
- Active phase (osteolytic phase)
  o Aggressive bone resorption with lytic lesions
  o Replacement of hematopoietic bone marrow by fibrous connective tissue
  o Increased vascular channels
- Inactive phase (quiescent phase)
  o Decreased bone turnover with skeletal sclerosis and coarse trabeculae
  o Loss of excessive vascularity
- Mixed pattern
  o Mixture of lytic and sclerotic phase

Clinical Issues
Presentation
- Age: 55-85 years, unusual <40 years, M:F=2:1
- Asymptomatic: 20%
- Fatigue
- Enlarged hat size
- Peripheral nerve compression, neurological disorders from compression of brainstem (basilar invagination)
- Sarcomatous transformation (< 1%)
- Compression fractures (soft bone despite increased density)
- Elevated serum alkaline phosphatase and urine hydroxyproline

Treatment & Prognosis
- Bisphosphates: Alendronate, etidronate
- Calcitonin

Selected References
1. Boutin RD et al: Complications in Paget disease at MR imaging. Radiology. 209:641-51, 1998
2. Roberts MC et al: Paget disease: MR imaging findings. Radiology. 173:341-5, 1989
3. Frame B et al: Paget disease: A review of current knowledge. Radiology. 141:21-4, 1981

BONE TUMORS

Osteoid Osteoma

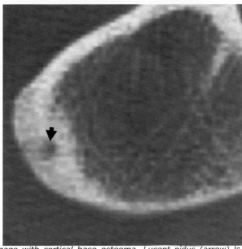

Axial CT image with cortical base osteoma. Lucent nidus (arrow) is epicentered within area of sclerotic cortical thickening.

Key Facts
- Represents 4% of primary bone tumors and 12% of benign bone tumors

Imaging Findings
General Features
- Meta-/ diaphysis of long bones (65%), femur and tibia (53%)
- Phalanges of hands and feet (21%)
- Spine (9%)
- Cortical (80%), intramedullary, intraarticular (preferentially hip)
MR Findings
- T1 MR: nidus isointense to muscle
- May have extensive bone marrow edema
- Synovitis and joint effusion with intra-articular lesion
CT Findings
- Study of choice for identifying nidus
- Small, well-defined, round/oval nidus surrounded by sclerosis
Plain Film Findings
- Radiolucent central nidus < 1.5 cm with surrounding sclerosis
- Periosteal reaction may be present
- Limb overgrowth in children if located near growth plate
Bone Scan Findings
- Increased uptake
- Double density sign: Small focus of increased activity (nidus) surrounded by larger area of less intense activity (reactive sclerosis)

Differential Diagnosis
Brodie's Abscess
- Linear, serpentine tract that extends away from abscess cavity
Bone Island
- No increased activity on bone scan

Osteoid Osteoma

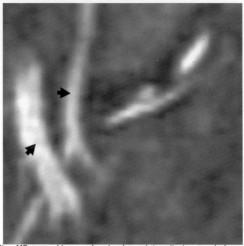

Corresponding MR coronal image showing hyperintensity in vessels (arrows) directed toward the nidus of osteoid osteoma (STIR coronal image).

Stress Fracture
- Radiolucency more linear and perpendicular to cortex (rather than parallel)

Pathology
General
- Etiology-Pathogenesis
  - Benign, highly vascular osteoblastic proliferation
  - Prostaglandin E2 elevated 100-1000 times within nidus (likely cause of pain and vasodilatation)

Gross Pathologic or Surgical Features
- Nidus: Less than 1 cm in greatest dimension
- Red/ tan mass of gritty osseous tissue
- Easily "shell out" from surrounding reactive bone

Microscopic Features
- Nidus composed of osteoid tissue or mineralized, immature, woven bone
- Osteoid matrix and bone form trabeculae surrounded by highly vascular, fibrous stroma with osteoblastic and osteoclastic activity
- Sclerosis surrounding lesion composed of dense bone

Clinical Issues
Presentation
- Age: 10-35 years, M:F=2:1
- Local pain worse at night, decreased by salicylates in less than 30 minutes (75%)
- Local swelling and point tenderness
- With spinal involvement painful scoliosis with concavity of curvature toward side of lesion

Osteoid Osteoma

Treatment & Prognosis
- Surgical resection of nidus
- Percutaneous radio-frequency ablation
- No growth progression, infrequent regression

Selected References
1.   Assoun J et al: Osteoid osteoma: MR imaging versus CT. Radiology. 191:217-23, 1994
2.   Azouz EM et al: Osteoid osteoma and osteoblastoma of the spine in children. Report of 22 cases with brief literature review. Pediatr Radiol. 16:25-31, 1986
3.   Cohen MD et al: Osteoid osteoma: 95 cases and a review of the literature. Semin Arthritis Rheum. 12:265-81, 1983

Osteoblastoma

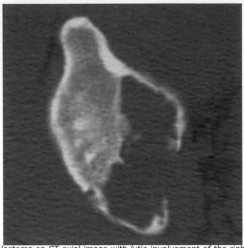

Osteoblastoma on CT axial image with lytic involvement of the right ilium.

Key Facts
- Represents <1% of all primary bone tumors
- Accounts for 3% of all benign bone tumors

Imaging Findings
General Features
- Spine: in posterior elements with secondary extension into vertebral body (40%)
- Long bones (30%)
- Hand and feet (15%)
- Skull and face (15%)
- Diaphyseal (58%), metaphyseal (42%)
- Eccentric (46%), intracortical (42%)

CT Findings
- Imaging modality of choice to demonstrate exact size and areas of ossification within lesion
- Aggressive osteoblastoma may disrupt cortex and have soft-tissue component

Plain Film Findings
- Expansile, well-circumscribed, lucent lesion
- Variable central calcification and matrix
- Rapidly increasing in size
- Cortical expansion (75-94%)/ destruction (20-22%)
- Radiolucent nidus >2cm
- No periosteal reaction

Bone Scan Findings
- Intense uptake

Differential Diagnosis
Osteoid Osteoma
- Smaller (<2 cm)
- Predilection for axial skeleton

Osteoblastoma

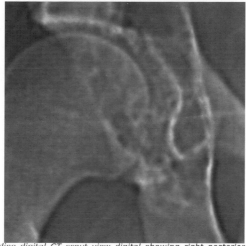

Corresponding digital CT scout view digital showing right posterior acetabular involvement with lytic osteoblastoma lesion.

- Tend toward regression while osteoblastoma tends toward progression
Osteosarcoma
- Periosteal new bone
- Soft-tissue component
Bone Abscess
- Serpentine tract extending toward growth plate
Aneurysmal Bone Cyst
- Fluid-fluid levels

Pathology
General
- General Path Comments
  - Lesion >1.5 cm, smaller lesions classified as osteoid osteoma
  - 10% recur after excision
Gross Pathologic or Surgical Features
- Well circumscribed and often surrounded by shell of cortical bone or periosteum
- Typically 2-10 cm, friable and deep red (high vascularity)
- Prominent cystic spaces may indicate secondary aneurysmal bone cyst formation
Microscopic Features
- Similar to osteoid osteoma with greater osteoid production and vascularity
- Numerous, multinucleated giant cells (osteoclasts)
- Very vascular connective tissue stroma with interconnecting trabecular bone

Clinical Issues
Presentation
- Age: 10-35 years, M:F=2:1
- Dull, localized pain of insidious onset, rarely interferes with sleep

Osteoblastoma

- Response to salicylates in 7%
- Localized swelling, tenderness, decreased range of motion
- Painful scoliosis with vertebral involvement

Treatment & Prognosis
- Surgical resection/excision of symptomatic lesions
- Radiation and chemotherapy in cases of aggressive and surgically unresectable lesions

Selected References
1. Della Rocca C et al: Osteoblastoma: Varied histological presentations with a benign clinical course. An analysis of 55 cases. Am J Surg Pathol. 20:841-50, 1996
2. Kroon HM et al: Osteoblastoma: Clinical and radiologic findings in 98 new cases. Radiology. 175:783-90, 1990

Enchondroma

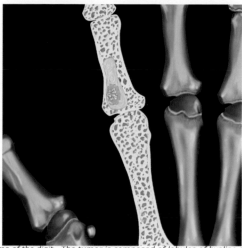

Enchondroma of the digit. The tumor is composed of lobules of hyaline cartilage and occasional flecks of calcifications.

Key Facts
- Second most common benign bone tumor
- Most common tumor of phalanges of the hand

Imaging Findings
General Features
- Any bone formed by enchondral ossification can be affected
- Short, tubular bones of hand and foot: 50%
- Femur, tibia, humerus, ribs: 50%
- Centrally located in diaphysis

Plain Film Findings
- Short, tubular bones: Radiolucent lesion
- Long bones: Chondroid calcification ("rings and arcs," "popcorn" appearance)
- Scalloped inner cortical margins
- Expansion of cortex without cortical break
- No periosteal reaction or soft-tissue mass
- Ollier disease: Non-hereditary failure of cartilage ossification
  - Multiple enchondromata
  - Predominantly unilateral monomelic distribution
  - Growth disparity with leg/arm shortening
  - Sarcomatous transformation in 25-50%: Osteosarcoma (young adults), chondrosarcoma/ fibrosarcoma (older patients)
- Maffucci syndrome: Non-hereditary multiple enchondromatosis and multiple soft-tissue cavernous hemangiomas
  - Unilateral involvement of hands and feet
  - Very large enchondromata, projecting into soft tissue
  - Phleboliths within hemangiomas
  - Malignant transformation of enchondroma into chondrosarcoma (15-25%)

Enchondroma

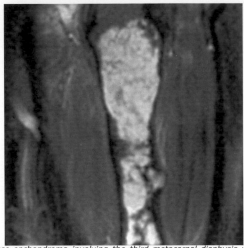

Hyperintense enchondroma involving the third metacarpal diaphysis with cortical breakthrough (FST2-FSE coronal image).

    o   Transformation of soft-tissue hemangioma into vascular sarcoma (3%)

<u>MR Findings</u>
- T1 MR: Low to intermediate SI
- T2 MR: High SI

Differential Diagnosis
<u>Bone Infarct</u>
- Well-defined, densely sclerotic, serpiginous borders
- No endosteal scalloping

<u>Chondrosarcoma</u>
- Clinical findings (primarily pain) better indicator of chondrosarcoma than radiographic findings
- Periosteal reaction, soft-tissue mass
- Size: > 4cm suggests malignancy

<u>Epidermoid Inclusion Cyst</u>
- Phalangeal tuft
- History of trauma

Pathology
<u>General</u>
- Etiology-Pathogenesis
  - o   Occurs in bones that form by enchondral ossification (not skull)
  - o   Develop from abnormal zone of dysplastic chondrocytes in growth plate which fail to undergo normal enchondral ossification
  - o   Rare malignant transformation of long bone enchondroma into chondrosarcoma

<u>Gross Pathologic or Surgical Features</u>
- Most enchondromas treated by curettage, resected specimens rare
- Tumor fragments consist of blue-white, glistering hyaline cartilage, sometimes mixed with yellow, calcified foci

- Resected tumors show focal lobules of mature hyaline cartilage ranging from millimeters to up to one centimeter in diameter

Microscopic Features

- Lobules of hyaline cartilage with translucent intercellular matrix (little collagen)
- Tumor cells located in lacunae
- Calcification common (correspond to matrix calcifications/ enchondral ossification)

Clinical Issues

Presentation

- Age: 15-40 years; peak age: 10-30 years, M:F=1:1
- Usually asymptomatic
- Painless swelling
- May present as pathologic fracture
- In absence of a fracture painful enchondroma is considered malignant until proven otherwise

Treatment & Prognosis

- Painful or worrisome lesions should be treated with biopsy followed by resection
- Large defects can be filled with bone graft

Selected References
1. Geirnaerdt MJ et al: Cartilaginous tumors: Correlation of gadolinium-enhanced MR imaging and histopathologic findings. Radiology. 186:813-7, 1993
2. Aoki J et al: MR of enchondroma and chondrosarcoma: Rings and arcs of Gd-DTPA enhancement. J Comput Assist Tomogr. 15:1011-6, 1991
3. Greenspan A: Tumors of cartilage origin. Orthop Clin North Am. 20:347-66, 1989

Osteochondroma

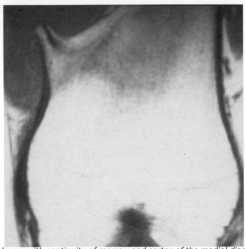

Osteochondroma with continuity of marrow and cortex of the medial diaphysis of the distal femur.

Key Facts
- Most common benign bone lesion
- Represents 45% of all benign bone tumors and 12% of all bone tumors

Imaging Findings
General Features
- Any bone with enchondromal ossification can be involved
- Metaphysis of femur, humerus, tibia (85%)

Plain Film Findings
- Cartilage covered bony projection (exostosis) on external surface of bone
- Continuity of bone cortex and medullary marrow space to host bone
- Pedunculated type: Slender pedicle directed away from joint
- Sessile type: Broad-based attachment to cortex
- Multiple hereditary osteochondromata: Autosomal-dominant hereditary disorder
  - Involves knee, hip, ankle, shoulder
  - Growth disturbance in forearm and leg
  - Sessile form more common
  - Increased risk of malignant transformation into chondrosarcoma

CT Findings
- To demonstrate continuity of cortical and medullary portions of lesion with host bone
- To demonstrate cartilaginous cap

MR Findings
- Cartilaginous cap high SI on T2

Differential Diagnosis
Malignant Transformation into Chondrosarcoma
- Development of thick, bulky, cartilaginous cap (thickness > 1cm by CT, >2cm by MRI)

Osteochondroma

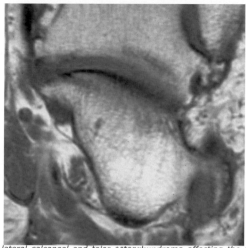

Prominent lateral calcaneal and talar osteochondroma affecting the ankle. Note hypointense signal from the associated bursa exostotica adjacent to the calcaneal osteochondroma (T1-weighted coronal image).

- Dispersed calcifications within cartilaginous cap
- Development of soft-tissue mass

Pathology
General
- General Path Comments
  - Lesions have own growth plate and stop growing with skeletal maturity
  - Malignant transformation into chondrosarcoma in <1% of solitary lesions

Gross Pathologic or Surgical Features
- Normal cortical bone with cartilaginous cap covered by thin, fibrous, periosteal layer
- Continuity of lesion with marrow and cortex of host bone (hallmark)

Microscopic Features
- Cartilage cap containing a basal surface with enchondral ossification
- Thickness of cap 1-3 mm, rarely up to 1 cm
- Greater thickness may imply malignant transformation

Clinical Issues
Presentation
- Age: 10-35 years, M:F=2:1
- Usually painless mass
- Painful with impingement of nerves/ blood vessels
- Malignant transformation into chondrosarcoma (< 1%)
  - Pain in absence of fracture, bursitis, nerve compression
  - Growth of lesion after skeletal maturation

Treatment & Prognosis
- Surgical resection of symptomatic lesions
- If entire cartilage cap removed recurrence unlikely

Osteochondroma

Selected References
1.   Karasick D et al: Symptomatic osteochondromas: Imaging features. AJR Am J Roentgenol. 168: 507-12, 1997
2.   Hudson TM et al: Benign exostoses and exostotic chondrosarcomas: Evaluation of cartilage thickness by CT. Radiology. 152:595-9, 1984

Chondroblastoma

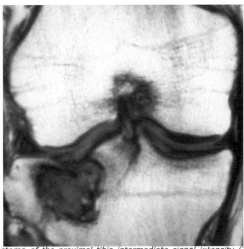

Chondroblastoma of the proximal tibia intermediate signal intensity (T1-weighted coronal Image).

Key Facts
- Represents <1% of all primary bone tumors and 9% of benign bone tumors

Imaging Findings

General Features
- Epiphysis of long bones (distal femur, proximal tibia, proximal humerus) or apophyses (greater trochanter of femur, patella, greater tuberosity of humerus)
- 2/3 in lower extremity, 50% about knee joint
- 20% involve flat bones or tubular bones of hands and feet
- May continue to involve metaphysis
- Usually seen in immature skeleton

Plain Film Findings
- Well-defined, eccentrically placed lytic lesion
- Thin sclerotic margin
- Geographic pattern of bone destruction
- Punctate/ irregular calcifications in 40-60%

MR Findings
- T2 MR: Intermediate to low heterogeneous SI
- Tends to overestimate extent and aggressiveness due to prominent soft tissue and bone marrow edema
- Joint effusions

Differential Diagnosis

Clear-Cell Chondrosarcoma
- May be indistinguishable
- Exhibits same benign pattern
- Both may be seen in immature skeleton

Giant Cell Tumor
- Usually larger and less well demarcated

Chondroblastoma

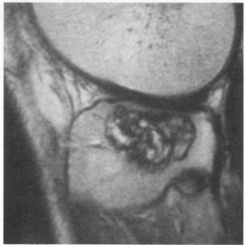

Inhomogeneity with hyperintense areas within chondroblastoma (T2-weighted sagittal).

- Not calcified
- Older age group with closed growth plate

Avascular Necrosis
- More irregular configuration
- Crescent sign

Pathology

General
- Etiology-Pathogenesis
  - Benign tumor that may become locally aggressive
  - Pulmonary metastases have been reported without histologic evidence of malignancy

Gross Pathology or Surgical Features
- Finely granular tumor with interspersed red areas (represent foci of hemorrhagic necrosis)
- Blue-gray areas correspond to chondroid matrix
- Larger tumors may break into metaphysis or through cortex

Microscopic Features
- Nodules of mature cartilage matrix surrounded by undifferentiated tissue of chondroblast-like cells
- "Chicken wire" calcification (pericellular deposition of calcification) pathognomonic

Clinical Issues

Presentation
- Peak age: 5-25 years, before cessation of enchondral bone growth
- M:F ratio = 2-3:1
- Mild joint pain, tenderness, swelling
- Joint effusion in 30%
- Pathologic fractures are rare

Chondroblastoma

<u>Treatment & Prognosis</u>
- Curettage with possible bone graft
- Excision of pulmonary nodules
- Recurrence in 25%

Selected References
1. Weatherall PT et al: Chondroblastoma: Classic and confusing appearance at MR imaging. Radiology 190:467-74, 1994
2. Bloem JL: Chondroblastoma: A clinical and radiological study of 104 cases. Skeletal Radiol 14:1-9, 1985

Non-Ossifying Fibroma

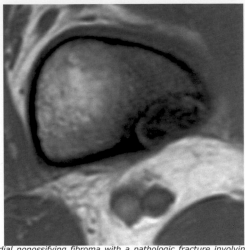

Posteromedial nonossifying fibroma with a pathologic fracture involving the distal femur. The non-ossifying fibroma is hypointense on T1-weighted axial images.

Key Facts
- Non-ossifying fibroma (NOF) and fibrous cortical defect (FCD) are histologically identical
- Most common fibrous lesion of bone
- Occurs in 20-30% of normal population during 1st and 2nd decades of life

Imaging Findings
General Features
- Involvement of tibia and fibula: 90%
- Metaphysis close to growth plate (postero-medially)
- Extending parallel to long axis of host bone
- Migrates toward center of diaphysis

Plain Film Findings
- Oval, radiolucent, cortical lesion with normal or thin sclerotic margins
- FCD: < 2, within the cortex
- NOF: > 2 cm, encroach on medullary cavity
- Resolve with age

MR Findings
- T1 ME: Low SI
- T2 MR: Low SI

Variants
- Jaffe-Campanacci syndrome: NOF with extraskeletal manifestations in children
  - Café-au-lait spots
  - Mental retardation
  - Cardiovascular congenital defect

Differential Diagnosis
Cortical Desmoid
- At tendinous insertion

Non-Ossifying Fibroma

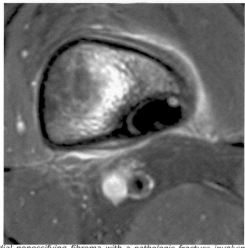

Posteromedial nonossifying fibroma with a pathologic fracture involving the distal femur. The non-ossifying fibroma is fat suppressed on T2-FSE axial images. A nonossifying fibroma may show increased or hypointense signal intensity on T2-weighted sequences.

Periosteal Reaction
Fibrous Dysplasia
- Expansile medullary lesion
- Ground glass appearance

Pathology
General
- Etiology Pathogenesis
    o Developmental defect arising in trabeculae of tubular bones and migrates toward diaphysis as bone grows in length
    o Involution over 2-4 years
    o Bone island in adult may be residue of incompletely involuted NOF
Gross Pathologic or Surgical Features
- Varying shades of gray and yellow, depending on relative proportions of fibrous tissue and foamy histiocytes
- Sharply rimmed by reactive bone
Microscopic Features
- Bundles of spindle-shaped fibroblasts and scattered, multinucleated giant cells and foamy histiocytes
- Arranged in a swirling pattern

Clinical Issues
Presentation
- Age: 2-20 years, M:F—2:1
- FCD: May cause pain, pathologic fracture
- NOF: Usually asymptomatic
- Hypophosphatemic vitamin D resistant rickets and osteomalacia (tumor may secrete substance that increases renal tubular resorption of phosphorus)

Non-Ossifying Fibroma

Treatment & Prognosis
- Surgery only in case of pathologic fractures

Selected References
1. Friedland JA et al: Quantitative analysis of the plain radiographic appearance of nonossifying fibroma. Invest Radiol. 30:474-9, 1995

Fibrous Dysplasia

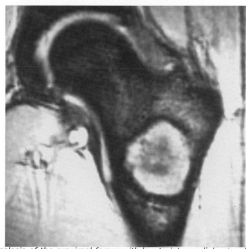

Fibrous dysplasia of the proximal femur with low to intermediate signal intensity In central area with peripheral increased signal intensity. The increase in fluid signal intensity is not as bright as fluid (T2* coronal image).

Key Facts
- Common developmental anomaly
- Most common benign lesion of the rib

Imaging Findings
General Features
- Involves metadiaphysis with sparing of epiphysis
- Monostotic form: 85%
  - Femoral neck, tibia, ribs, base of skull
- Polyostotic form: 15%
  - Pelvis, long bones, skull, ribs
  - Unilateral or monomelic

Plain Film Findings
- Radiolucent, expansile, medullary lesion
- Ground glass appearance
- Well-defined sclerotic margins, endosteal scalloping
- No periostits
- Frontal bossing, facial asymmetry
- Bowing deformities of long bones (shepherd's crook deformity)

Bone Scan Findings
- To determine activity and extent of involvement
- Increased uptake in majority of lesions

Variants
- Cherubism: Symmetric involvement of mandible and maxilla
  - Autosomal dominant
- McCune Albright syndrome: Polyostotic unilateral fibrous dysplasia
  - Endocrine abnormalities (precocious puberty, hyperthyroidism)
  - Café-au-lait spots ("Coast of Maine")
  - Female predominance

Fibrous Dysplasia

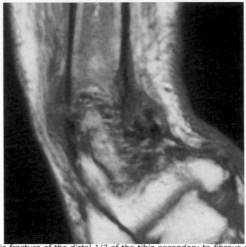

Pathologic fracture of the distal 1/3 of the tibia secondary to fibrous dysplasia.

- Mazabraud syndrome: Multiple, fibrous, soft-tissue tumors in association with polyostotic fibrous dysplasia
- Leontiasis ossea (craniofacial fibrous dysplasia)
  o Involvement of facial and frontal bones
  o Leonine facies (resembling a lion)
  o Cranial nerve palsies

Differential Diagnosis
Neurofibromatosis
- Long-bone deformities without intramedullary changes
Paget's Disease
- Radiographically identical to monostotic cranial lesion
Osteofibrous Dysplasia
- Almost exclusively in tibia of infants
- Lesion begins in cortex
Enchondroma
- Lesions may extend into articular ends of bones

Pathology
General
- Etiology-Pathogenesis
  o Benign developmental abnormality in which medullary cavity is replaced with fibrous tissue that contains immature woven bone
  o Probable gene mutation during embryogenesis
  o Does not spread, proliferate
  o Malignant transformation is rare (0.5%)
Gross Pathologic or Surgical Features
- Firm, fibrous, white or red tissue with variable gritty consistency, depending on the amount of mineralized bone
- Secondary blood-filled cyst formation common

Fibrous Dysplasia

Microscopic Features
- Medullary cavity replaced by immature matrix of collagen with small, irregularly-shaped trabeculae of immature "woven" bone and inadequate mineralization
- Low-power photomicrographic picture: Alphabet soup

Clinical Issues
Presentation
- Age: 5-50 years; peak age: 10-20 years, M:F=1:1
- Monostotic form: Usually asymptomatic
  o Can present with pathologic fracture
- Polyostotic form: 2/3 symptomatic by age 10
  o Leg pain, limp, pathologic fracture
  o Abnormal vaginal bleeding (25%)
  o Endocrine disorders: Hyperthyroidism, hyperparathyroidism, McCune Albright syndrome (precocious puberty)
- Soft-tissue myxomas

Treatment & Prognosis
- Surgery not necessary for asymptomatic lesions unless bone is at risk for pathologic fracture
- Surgery with curettage associates with high rate of local recurrence

Selected References
1. Choi KH et al: Fibrous dysplasia: MR imaging characteristics with radiopathologic correlation. AJR Am J Roentgenol. 167:1523-7, 1996
2. Inamo Y et al: Findings on magnetic resonance imaging of the spine and femur in a case of McCune-Albright syndrome. Pediatr Radiol.23:15-8, 1993
3. Utz JA et al: MR appearance of fibrous dysplasia. J Comput Assist Tomogr. 13:845-51, 1989

Unicameral Bone Cyst

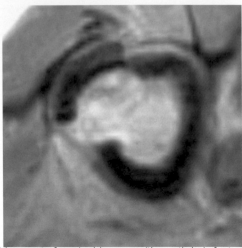

Unicameral bone cyst of proximal humerus with a pathologic fracture. Lesion is intermediate in signal intensity on proton density.

Key Facts
- Represent 3% of primary bone lesions

Imaging Findings
General Features
- Proximal metaphysis of humerus and femur (60-75%)
- Calcaneus, talus, ilium (50%): In older patients
- Adjacent to epiphyseal cartilage (during active phase)
- Migrating into diaphysis with growth (during latent phase) without crossing growth plate

Plain Film Findings
- Centrally located, well-circumscribed, expansile, lucent lesion with sclerotic margins
- Scalloping of underlying cortex
- Fluid-filled cavity (fluid/ fluid levels)
- No periosteal reaction unless fractured
- Fallen fragment sign secondary to pathologic fracture (pathognomonic): Fragment migrates to dependent portions of cyst

Differential Diagnosis
Aneurysmal Bone Cyst
- Eccentric lesion with periosteal reaction
- Geographic type of bone destruction

Fibrous Dysplasia
- No trabeculation
- Ground glass, smoky appearance

Brown Tumor/ Hyperparathyroidism
- Other features of hyperparathyroidism (osteopenia and subcortical resorption)

Bone Abscess
- Periosteal reaction

Unicameral Bone Cyst

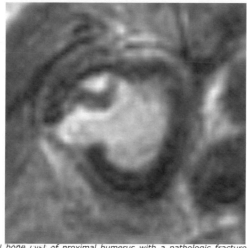

Unicameral bone cyst of proximal humerus with a pathologic fracture. Lesion is hyperintense on T2-weighted axial image.

- Extension beyond boundaries of growth plate

Pathology
General
- Etiology-Pathogenesis
  - Tumor-like lesion of unknown cause, attributed to local disturbance of bone growth
  - Appears to be reactive or developmental rather than neoplastic

Gross Pathologic or Surgical Features
- Intact specimens rarely seen
- Curetted fragments contain serous yellow fluid
- Wall of cyst is white and shiny and 1 mm thick

Microscopic Features
- Wall of cavity lined with fibrous tissue or granulation tissue containing hemosiderin deposits and small lymphocyte infiltrates
- Membrane contains giant cells of osteoclastic type
- Fluid usually shows elevated alkaline phosphatase
- Spontaneous regression in majority of cases

Clinical Issues
Presentation
- Age: 10-20 years, M:F=3:1
- 66% of cysts present with pathologic fractures and pain

Treatment & Prognosis
- Percutaneous injection of corticosteroids
- Open curettage with bone graft has high recurrence rate

Selected References
1. Kransdorf MJ et al: Aneurysmal bone cyst: concept, controversy, clinical presentation, and imaging. AJR Am J Roentgenol. 164:573-80, 1995
2. Conway WF et al: Miscellaneous lesions of bone. Radiol Clin North Am. 31:339-58, 1993
3. Struhl S et al: Solitary (unicameral) bone cyst. The fallen fragment sign revisited. Skeletal Radiol. 18:261-5, 1989

Giant Cell Tumor

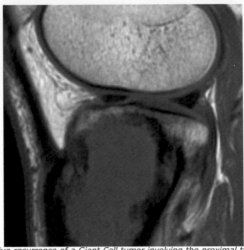

Postoperative recurrence of a Giant Cell tumor involving the proximal tibia. Tumor is hypointense on T1 image.

Key Facts
- Represents 5% of all primary bone tumors
- Sixth most common primary bone tumor

Imaging Findings
General Features
- Within epiphysis at the articular surface of long bones (85%)
- Flat bones (15%): Pelvis, sacrum near SI joint

Plain Film Findings
- Expansile, solitary, lytic bone lesion ("soap bubble" appearance)
- Eccentrically located with well-defined borders
- Conspicuous peripheral trabeculae without tumor matrix
- No sclerosis/ periosteal reaction

CT Findings
- Tumor of soft-tissue attenuation with foci of low attenuation (hemorrhage/necrosis)
- May break through bone cortex with cortical thinning, soft-tissue invasion

MR Findings
- T1 MR: Low to intermediate SI, best to see intramedullary portion of tumor
- T2 MR: High SI, best to see extraosseous component of tumor
- Fluid-fluid levels

Bone Scan Findings
- "Doughnut" sign: Intense uptake around periphery with little activity in central portions of tumor
- May help in detection of multicentric giant cell tumor

Differential Diagnosis
Aneurysmal Bone Cyst
- Rarely affects articular end of bone

Giant Cell Tumor

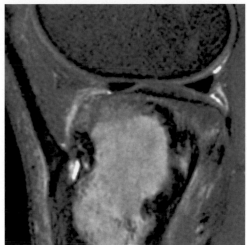

Postoperative recurrence of a Giant Cell tumor involving the proximal tibia. Tumor is hyperintense on FST2-FSE image.

- Younger age group
- May coexist with giant cell tumor

Brown Tumor
- Accompanied by other skeletal manifestations (osteomalacia, cortical/subperiosteal resorption)

Chondroblastoma
- Calcified
- Younger age group

Intraosseous Ganglion
- Sclerotic border

Pathology
General
- General Path Comments
  - Locally aggressive, 12-50% recurrence rate
  - Clinical behavior cannot be predicted on basis of radiological and histologic features
  - Can undergo sarcomatous transformation, spontaneously or in response to radiation therapy
  - Pulmonary metastases in 1-2% that are histologically identical to primary tumor
  - 0.5-1% multifocal, associated with Paget disease

Gross Pathologic or Surgical Features
- Can be hemorrhagic (resemble aneurysmal bone cyst) or soft and fleshy
- In long bones tumor abuts articular cartilage
- Surrounding bone is expanded with thinning of the cortex

Microscopic Features
- Multinucleated osteoclastic giant cells intermixed throughout a spindle cell stroma
- Osteoclastic giant cells not apposed to bone surfaces, do not participate in bone resorption

Giant Cell Tumor

Clinical Issues
Presentation
- Age range: 20-40 years, occurs after skeletal maturity
- F:M=2:1
- Pain and swelling at affected area
- Pathologic fracture in 30%

Treatment & Prognosis
- Surgical resection with bone graft/ filling of cavity with cement
- Curettage alone associated with high rate of recurrence
- Wide excision in cases with recurrence
- Radiation only for cases of unresectable tumor due to sarcomatous degeneration
- Prognosis related to destruction of adjacent joint

Selected References
1. Schutte HE et al: Giant cell tumor in children and adolescents. Skeletal Radiol. 22:173-6, 1993
2. Aoki J et al: Giant cell tumors of bone containing large amounts of hemosiderin: MR-pathologic correlation. J Comput Assist Tomogr. 15:1024-7, 1991
3. Carrasco CH et al: Giant cell tumors. Orthop Clin North Am. 20:395-405, 1989

Osteosarcoma

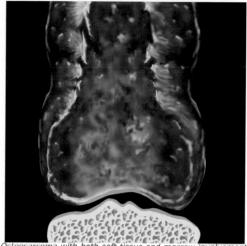

Osteosarcoma with both soft tissue and marrow involvement.

Key Facts
- Most common malignant primary bone tumor in young adults and children
- Second most common primary malignant bone tumor

Imaging Findings
General Features
- Metaphyses of long tubular bones (80%), 55% around knee
- Flat bones, vertebral bodies (20%)
- Extension into epiphysis (75%)

Plain Film Findings
- Primary osseous osteosarcoma (95%)
  - Conventional OSA
    - Poorly-defined, intramedullary mass, extends through cortex
    - Moth-eaten bone destruction
    - Aggressive periosteal reaction: Codman triangle, sunburst pattern
    - Indistinct borders with wide zone of transition
  - Telangiectatic osteosarcoma
    - Very malignant, worst prognosis
    - Purely lytic lesion
    - Cystic cavities filled with blood/ necrosis
    - Fluid levels (may mimic ABC)
  - Multicentric osteosarcoma
    - Synchronous osteoblastic osteosarcoma at multiple sites (usually symmetric)
    - Exclusively in children (5-10 years)
    - Extremely poor prognosis
- Juxtacortical osteosarcoma
  - Periosteal osteosarcoma
    - Low grade osteosarcoma in older age group (20-50 years)
    - Posterior distal femur

Osteosarcoma

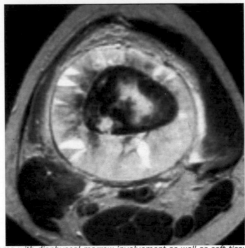

Osteosarcoma with diaphyseal marrow involvement as well as soft tissue extension (T2-weighted axial image).

- ▪ Attached to underlying cortex at origin
  - o Periosteal osteosarcoma (extremely rare)
    - ▪ Intermediate-grade osteosarcoma
    - ▪ Most common diaphyseal
    - ▪ No medullary involvement
    - ▪ Cortical thickening
- Secondary osteosarcoma
  - o Arises in association with preexisting lesion of bone such as Paget disease, prior radiation, dedifferentiated chondrosarcoma, or bone infarct

MR Findings
- To determine extent of tumor within bone marrow and soft tissue, relationship to vessels and nerves
- T1 MR: Low SI (mineralized tumor), low-intermediate SI (solid, non-mineralized tumor)
- T2 MR: Low SI (mineralized tumor), high SI (non-mineralized tumor, soft tissue mass)

Bone Scan Findings
- For staging
- Detection of skip lesions, metastases

Differential Diagnosis
Ewing Sarcoma
- Diaphysis of long bones
- Large soft-tissue mass
Clear Cell Chondrosarcoma
- Both can involve epiphysis
Fibrous Dysplasia
- Expansive lesion with thinned cortex
- Narrow zone of transition
- No cortical destruction or periosteal reactions

Osteosarcoma

Pathology
Under<u>General</u>
- Etiology-Pathogenesis
  - Malignant tumor with ability to produce osteoid directly from neoplastic cells

<u>Gross Pathologic or Surgical Features</u>
- White-tan, firm, gritty mass with foci of hemorrhage and necrosis
- Penetration of cortex with often large extraosseous tumor mass
- Periosteal reaction visible as lamellae of new bone at periphery of lesion

<u>Microscopic Features</u>
- Highly pleomorphic, spindle-shaped tumor cells producing different forms of osteoid
- Three histologic subtypes depending on sarcomatous component: Osteoblastic, chondroblastic, fibroblastic osteosarcoma

Clinical Issues
<u>Presentation</u>
- Age: 10-30 years, M≥F,
- Pain, development of soft-tissue swelling or mass, fever
- Pulmonary metastases common, can cause pneumothorax (calcifying)

<u>Treatment & Prognosis</u>
- Adjuvant and neoadjuvant chemotherapy and surgical resection
- Prognosis dependent on osteosarcoma type, size, location, and presence of metastases

Selected References
1. Rosenberg ZS et al: Osteosarcoma: Subtle, rare, and misleading plain film features. AJR Am J Roentgenol. 165:1209-14, 1995
2. Mervak TR et al: Telangiectatic osteosarcoma. Clin Orthop. 270:135-9, 1991
3. Sundaram M et al: Magnetic resonance imaging of osteosarcoma. Skeletal Radiol. 16:23-9, 1987

Chondrosarcoma

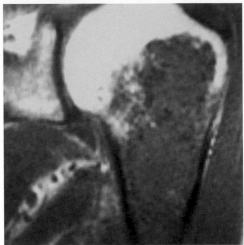

Chondrosarcoma with hypointense calcifications within the chondroid matrix of the tumor. The tumor itself is hypointense to intermediate in signal intensity on T1-weighted coronal image.

Key Facts
- Third most common primary malignant bone tumor
- Represents 10% of all primary bone sarcomas

Imaging Findings
General Features
- Involves the flat bones (pelvis)
- Meta-/ diaphysis of long bones (especially femur)
- May extend into epiphysis

Plain Film Findings
- Lytic mass with or without chondroid matrix
- Medullary (central) chondrosarcoma (80% of cases)
  - Expansion of medullary cavity
  - Thickening of cortex with endosteal scalloping
  - Popcorn-like calcification
  - May present with large soft-tissue mass
- Exostotic (peripheral) chondrosarcoma
  - Malignant degeneration of hereditary multiple exostoses
  - Can arise in cartilage cap of a previously benign osteochondroma
  - Thickening of cortex and soft-tissue mass at site of attachment to bone
  - Chondroid matrix
  - Late destruction of bone
- Dedifferentiated chondrosarcoma
  - Ill-defined, lytic lesion in continuity with cartilaginous tumor
  - Abrupt transition between cartilaginous tumor and dedifferentiated lytic component
- Clear cell chondrosarcoma
  - Round, sharply-marginated, lytic lesion in epiphysis of long bones
  - May contain calcifications

Chondrosarcoma

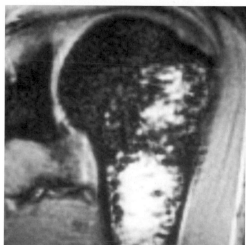

Corresponding hyperintense chondroid matrix with hypointense calcifications within medullary chondrosarcoma (T2* coronal image).

- o Surrounding sclerosis
- o Indistinguishable from chondroblastoma (slow growth over years)
- Extraskeletal chondrosarcoma
  - o 2% of all soft-tissue sarcomas
  - o Extremities, particularly thigh most common
  - o Lobulated soft-tissue mass with and without calcification

MR Findings
- To determine intramedullary extent and soft-tissue invasion
- T1 MR: Low to intermediate SI
- T2 M: High SI and low SI areas (represent mineralization)

CT Findings
- Chondroid matrix mineralization of "rings and arcs" (characteristic)
- Nonmineralized portions of tumor hypodense to muscle (high water content of hyaline cartilage)

Differential Diagnosis
Enchondroma
- No periosteal reaction and cortical destruction
- No soft-tissue mass
- Development of pain and swelling in previously asymptomatic enchondroma suspicious for malignant degeneration

Chondroblastoma
- May be indistinguishable from clear cell chondrosarcoma
- Both occur in epiphyses and can occur before skeletal maturity

Pathology
General
- Etiology-Pathogenesis
  - o Malignant tumor in which neoplastic cells form cartilage but not osteoid

Chondrosarcoma

- o Can occur as primary chondrosarcoma or as malignant degeneration of osteochondroma or enchondroma
- o Degeneration into fibrosarcoma, MFH, or osteosarcoma in 10%
- o Metastases (uncommon) to lung

Gross Pathologic or Surgical Features
- Consistency of hyaline cartilage with translucent blue-gray color
- Hemorrhagic necrosis especially in high-grade tumors
- Central lesions erode and eventually destroy cortex with extension into surrounding soft tissue

Microscopic Features
- Irregular-shaped lobules of cartilage
- May be separated by narrow, fibrous bands
- Chondrocytes arranged in clusters, can be mononuclear or multinucleated
- Matrix: Mature hyaline cartilage or myxoid stroma

Clinical Issues

Presentation
- Age 20-90 years, peak age: 40-60 years, M:F=2:1
- Pain with or without mass
- Pathologic fractures rare
- Pelvic chondrosarcoma may invade bladder or colon

Treatment & Prognosis
- Wide surgical excision
- Limited role for chemotherapy or radiation therapy
- Biopsies must be planned with future tumor excision in mind
- Patients with adequately resected, low-grade chondrosarcomas have excellent survival rate
- The survival of patients with high-grade tumors depends on the location, size, and stage of the tumor

Selected References
1. West OC et al: Quantitative analysis of the plain radiographic appearance of central chondrosarcoma of bone. Invest Radiol. 30:440-7, 1995
2. Mercuri M et al: Dedifferentiated chondrosarcoma. Skeletal Radiol. 24:409-16, 1995
3. Aoki J et al: MR of enchondroma and chondrosarcoma: Rings and arcs of Gd-DTPA enhancement. J Comput Assist Tomogr. 15:1011-6, 1991

Ewing's Sarcoma

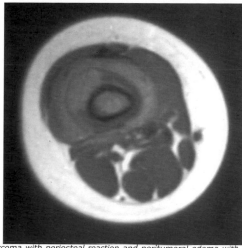

Ewing's sarcoma with periosteal reaction and peritumoral edema with marrow and soft-tissue extension (T1-weighted axial image).

Key Facts
- Represents 11-12% of all bone tumors
- Sixth most common malignant bone tumor

Imaging Findings
General Features
- Diaphysis of long bones: 70%
- Flat bones (sacrum, scapula): 25%
- Vertebral body: 5%

Plain Film Findings
- Ill-defined, lytic lesion with permeative/ moth eaten bone destruction
- Cortical erosion with "onion skin" or "sunburst" periosteal reaction, Codman triangle
- Penetration into soft tissue with extraosseous, non-calcified, soft-tissue mass (50%)
- No tumor matrix

MR Findings
- To assess extent of intra-and extraosseous involvement
- T1 MR: Intermediate to low SI
- T2 MR: High SI
- Enhancement of Gd-DTPA in cellular areas (to differentiate tumor from peritumoral edema)

Bone Scan Findings
- For evaluation of skeletal metastases
- Intense uptake of 99m Tc-MDP
- Gallium-67-citrate scan to determine soft-tissue extension

Differential Diagnosis
Osteomyelitis
- May look identical
- Duration of symptoms usually more sensitive

Ewing's Sarcoma

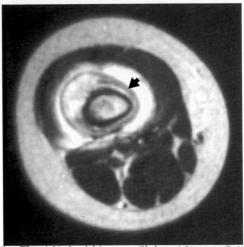

Corresponding T2-weighted axial images with hyperintense peritumoral edema superficial to periosteal reaction (arrow). The soft-tissue and marrow involvement are hyperintense (T2-weighted axial image).

Eosinophilic Granuloma
- Solid periosteal reaction

Osteosarcoma
- Usually involves metaphyses
- Bone formation within destructive lesion and soft tissue

Lymphoma
- Older age group
- Absence of soft-tissue mass

Primitive Neuroectodermal Tumor (PNET)
- Can not be differentiated from Ewing's sarcoma on basis of radiography

Metastatic Neuroblastoma
- Patients younger than 5 years

Pathology
General
- Etiology-Pathogenesis
  - Derived from undifferentiated mesenchymal cells of the bone marrow or primitive neuroectodermal cells (small round cell tumor)
  - Clinically, radiologically, and histologically very similar to PNET

Gross Pathologic or Surgical Features
- Intraosseous component: Firm, gray-white, moist mass
- Extraosseous component: Softer and more friable, may be considerably larger than intraosseous tumor

Microscopic Features
- Densely packed, small, uniform cells with round nuclei invading medullary cavity
- Clear cytoplasm and nuclei with prominent cytoplasmic glycogen
- No microscopic evidence of matrix production

Ewing's Sarcoma

Clinical Issues
Presentation
- Age: 5-25 years; peak age: 15 years, M:F=2:1, Caucasians: 96%
- Severe localized pain
- Soft-tissue mass
- Fever, leukocytosis, elevated ESR simulating osteomyelitis (indicated disseminated disease)
- Metastases to lung, regional lymph nodes, and other bones in 30% at presentation
- Pathologic fractures uncommon

Treatment & Prognosis
- Resection, radiation therapy, adjuvant and neoadjuvant chemotherapy
- Poor prognostic signs include increased age, increased ESR and leukocytosis at presentation

Selected References
1. Eggli KD et al: Ewing's sarcoma. Radiol Clin North Am. 31:325-37, 1993
2. Oestreich AE: Imaging of the skeleton and soft tissues in children. Curr Opin Radiol. 4:55-61, 1992
3. Boyko OB et al: MR imaging of osteogenic and Ewing's sarcoma. AJR Am J Roentgenol. 148:317-22, 1987

PocketRadiologist™
Musculoskeletal
100 Top Diagnoses

SOFT TISSUE TUMORS

Fibromatosis

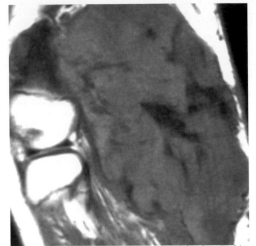

Desmoid tumor with fibrous stroma on T1-weighted sagittal image.

Key Facts
- Variety of benign disorders with fibrous growth and tendency to infiltrate adjacent tissues and to recur

Imaging Findings
General Features
- Involves superficial fasciae, deep tendons, aponeuroses, muscles
- Shoulder, upper arm, thigh, neck, pelvis, abdomen, forearm

CT Findings
- Hyperdense to muscle
- Intense contrast enhancement
- If close proximity to bone: Erosion, cortical destruction, periosteal reaction

MR Findings
- Poorly defined (with invasion of fat/muscle)
- T1 MR: Iso-hypointense to muscle
- T2 MR: High SI with areas of low SI (fibrous components)

US Findings
- Variable echogenicity
- Smooth, well-defined margins

Differential Diagnosis
MFH
- Arises in deep soft tissues
- Calcifications

Synovial Sarcoma
- In close proximity to joint
- Amorphous calcifications

Fibromatosis

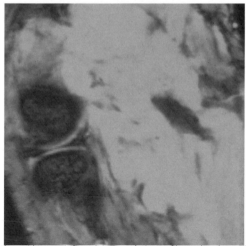

Soft tissue desmoid tumor is hyperintense relative to fibrous bands on T2* weighted sagittal image. The fibrous band or stroma is hypointense.

Pathology
General
- General Path Comments
  - Despite capacity for locally aggressive infiltrative behavior and recurrence self-limited disease, incapable of metastasizing

Gross Pathologic or Surgical Features
- Firm, gray-white mass with streaky, scar-like cross section
- May appear well circumscribed but microscopically have ill-defined borders

Microscopic Features
- Proliferation of uniform fibroblastic cells, accompanied by abundant, dense, collagenous stroma
- Resembling hypertrophic scar tissue

Clinical Issues
Presentation
- Age: 20-40 years; peak age: 23 years, M=F
- Tender and painful soft-tissue mass

Treatment & Prognosis
- Surgical excision
- Radiation therapy in aggressive, recurrent lesions

Selected References
1. Liu P et al: MRI of fibromatosis: With pathologic correlation. Pediatr Radiol. 22:587-9, 1992
2. O'Keefe F, et al: Magnetic resonance imaging in aggressive fibromatosis. Clin Radiol. 42:170-3, 1990
3. Hudson TM et al: Aggressive fibromatosis: Evaluation by computed tomography and angiography. Radiology. 150:495-501, 1984

Lipoma

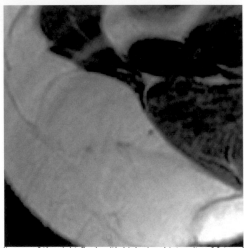

Soft-tissue lipoma of the right flank with high signal intensity of fat on T1-weighted axial image.

Key Facts
- Most common soft-tissue tumor

Imaging Findings
General Features
- Superficial/ subcutaneous lipoma (most common): Posterior trunk, neck, proximal extremities
- Deep lipoma: Retroperitoneum, chest wall, deep soft-tissue of hands and feet
- Multiple in 5-7%

CT Findings
- Well-defined and homogeneous tumor with low attenuation (-65 to 120 HU)
- Very variable size
- No enhancement following IV contrast
- Occasional ossification within tumor
- May cause cortical thickening when located close to bone

MR Findings
- T1 MR: High SI
- T2 MR: Intermediate SI
- Well defined and homogeneous, often with septations
- Differentiation from other lesions by fat suppression
- Intramuscular lipoma may be poorly marginated and infiltrate muscle planes

Differential Diagnosis
Liposarcoma
- Inhomogeneous mass with fat and soft-tissue components
- Enhancement after IV contrast administration

Lipoma

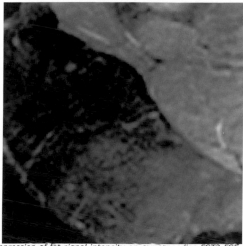

Uniform suppression of fat signal intensity on corresponding FST2-FSE axial image.

Pathology
<u>General</u>
- General Path Comments
  - Tumor tissue similar to ordinary body fat
  - Fat unavailable for systemic metabolism in cases of starvation

<u>Gross Pathologic or Surgical Features</u>
- Soft, well-encapsulated, lobulated mass consisting of yellow, grossly normal-appearing fat

<u>Microscopic Features</u>
- Mature, uniform fat cells (adipocytes)
- Fibrous connective tissue as septations

Clinical Issues
<u>Presentation</u>
- Age: 5-75 years; peak age: 50-60 years, F>M
- Asymptomatic lesion

<u>Treatment & Prognosis</u>
- Marginal excision of large lesions
- Recurrence is rare

Selected References
1. Gelineck J et al: Evaluation of lipomatous soft tissue tumors by MR imaging. Acta Radiol. 35:367-70, 1994
2. Roth D et al: Adipose tumors of soft tissues. J Belge Radiol. 75:371-6, 1992

Neurofibroma

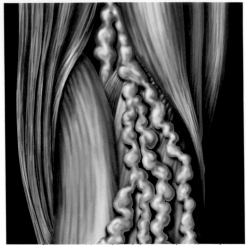

Plexiform neurofibromas with multinodular growth pattern demonstrated.

Key Facts
- Benign lesion of neural origin that may occur in peripheral nerves, soft tissue, skin, or bone

Imaging Findings
General Features
- May form in neural plexus, peripheral, or spinal nerve
- Solitary in 90%, most often involvement of cutaneous nerves
- Multiple tumors: Associated with neurofibromatosis type 1 (NF-1), non-cutaneous nerves often involved

MR Findings
- Peripheral nerve involvement
  - Non-encapsulated well-circumscribed fusiform mass
- Intradural extramedullary mass
  - Well-defined mass with dumbbell configuration (extradural component extends through neural foramen)
  - Widening of intervertebral foramina
  - Erosion of pedicles
  - Scalloping of vertebral bodies
  - Usually no contrast enhancement
  - T1 MR: Isointense to muscle
  - T2 MR: Hyperintense compared to surrounding fat
  - "Target Sign": Low SI center (due to collagen and condensed Schwann cells)

Differential Diagnosis
Schwannoma
- Involvement of cranial nerve VIII common
- T1 MR: 70% hypointense, 30% isointense to muscle
- Commonly associated with NF-2
- Dense enhancement

Neurofibroma

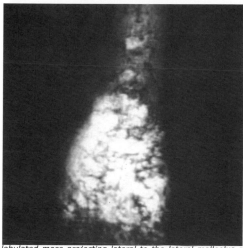

Soft-tissue lobulated mass projecting lateral to the lateral malleolus of the ankle. This soft-tissue mass has the lobulated, hyperintense contour characteristic of plexiform neurofibromatosis. Tumor is hyperintense on T2* weighted sagittal image.

Pathology
General
- General Path Comments
  - Associated with NF-1, however only 10% of patients with neurofibromas have NF-1

Gross Pathologic or Surgical Features
- Firm, gray-white mass without capsule
- Solitary neurofibromas: Well delineated and firm, white, shiny appearance
- Plexiform neurofibromas: Multifocal myxoid lesions, "bag of worms," diagnostic of NF-1
- Size ranges from few millimeters to four to five centimeters

Microscopic Features
- Tumor of nerve sheath, composed of interlacing bundles of Schwann cells, fibroblasts, with involvement of nerve fibers
- Immunoreactivity: Variable S-100 expression

Clinical Issues
Presentation
- Age: 20-30 years
- Superficial, painless mass in the dermis
- Potential for malignant transformation: Rare in solitary tumor, 4% in NF-1
- Associated with NF-1: Neurofibromas, acoustic nerve schwannomas, Lisch nodules, café-au-lait spots

Treatment & Prognosis
- Surgical excision of symptomatic lesions

Neurofibroma

Selected References
1. Beggs I: Pictorial review: Imaging of peripheral nerve tumors. Clin Radiol. 52:8-17, 1997
2. Pollack IF et al: Neurofibromatosis 1 and 2. Brain Pathol. 7:823-36, 1997

Liposarcoma

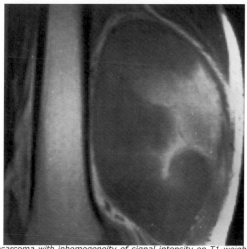

Myxoid liposarcoma with inhomogeneity of signal intensity on T1-weighted sagittal image. There are hypo and hyperintense areas visualized.

Key Facts
- Represents 20% of all malignant soft-tissue tumors
- 2nd most common soft-tissue sarcoma in adults

Imaging Findings
General Features
- Trunk (42%)
- Lower extremity (41%), upper extremity (11%)
- Head and neck (6%)
CT Findings
- Inhomogeneous soft-tissue mass of variable size (5cm -> 30cm)
- Fat frequently radiologically not detectable
- Occasionally ossification within tumor
- Enhancement after IV contrast
MR Findings
- Fat may or may not be present
- T1 MR: Hypointense
- T2 MR: Hyperintense

Differential Diagnosis
Lipoma
- Homogeneous soft-tissue mass
- No enhancement after IV contrast administration

Pathology
General
- Malignant tumor of mesenchymal origin with fat-forming cells (lipoblasts)
- Biologic behavior and prognosis determined by histologic type
Gross Pathologic or Surgical Features
- Well-circumscribed, lobular tumor with smooth surface

251

Liposarcoma

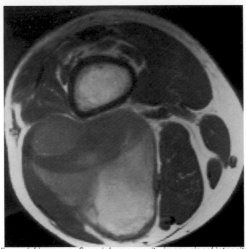

Corresponding axial image confirms inhomogeneity image signal intensity with areas of increased signal intensity representing the lipomatous portion of the tumor (T1-weighted axial image).

- Color and consistency varies with histologic composition (from soft, bright yellow to fleshy, firm with large areas of necrosis and hemorrhage)

Microscopic Features
- Well-differentiated type (15%): Best prognosis, composed of large, mature lipocytes with varying degrees of nuclear atypia
- Myxoid type (40-50%): Proliferating fibroblasts, plexiform capillary pattern, myxoid matrix, fat amount < 10%
- Round cell type (<10%): Poorly differentiated, highly cellular tumor, composed of primitive, small, round cells with sporadic lipoblastic differentiation, areas of hemorrhage and necrosis common
- Pleomorphic type (25%): Highly anaplastic tumor, pleomorphic cells growing in disorderly fashion, voluminous cytoplasm filled with lipid vacuoles which displace and distort nuclei ("scalloped" effect)

Clinical Issues
Presentation
- Age: 50-60 years, M>F
- Usually painless mass (Painful in 10-15%)
- Metastases to lung, visceral organs

Treatment & Prognosis
- Surgical resection with wide margins
- Resection and radiation therapy in selected cases
- Prognosis dependent on cell type: Pleomorphic type worst prognosis

Selected References
1. Arkun R et al: Liposarcoma of soft tissue: MRI findings with pathologic correlation. Skeletal Radiol. 26:167-72, 1997
2. Crim JR et al: Diagnosis of soft-tissue masses with MR imaging: Can benign masses be differentiated from malignant ones? Radiology. 185:581-6, 1992.
3. Sundaram M et al: Myxoid liposarcoma: Magnetic resonance imaging appearances with clinical and histological correlation. Skeletal Radiol. 19:359-62, 1990.

Malignant Fibrous Histiocytoma

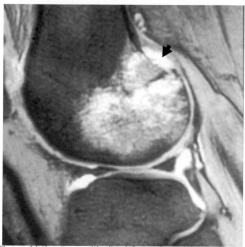

Malignant fibrous histiocytoma with distal femoral condylar involvement showing posterior cortical (arrow) breakthrough (T2 sagittal image).*

Key Facts
- Most common primary malignant soft-tissue tumor of late adult life
- 20-30% of all soft-tissue sarcomas
- Clinically and radiographically indistinguishable from fibrosarcoma

Imaging Findings
General Features
- Large muscle groups of extremities: 75%,
  - Lower extremity: 50%, upper extremity: 25%
- Deep soft tissues of retroperitoneum: 15%
- Head and neck: 5%
- Chest wall

Plain Film Findings
- Soft-tissue mass with poorly defined, curvilinear/ punctate peripheral calcifications
- Cortical erosions of adjacent bone

CT Findings
- Well-defined soft-tissue mass with central hypodense area
- Enhancement of solid components

MR Findings
- Inhomogeneous, poorly-defined lesion
- T1 MR: Low SI
- T2 MR: High SI

Differential Diagnosis
Liposarcoma
- Younger patients
- Presence of fat in > 40%
- Calcifications rare

Synovial Sarcoma
- Cortical erosions

Malignant Fibrous Histiocytoma

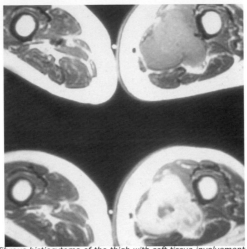

Malignant fibrous histiocytoma of the thigh with soft tissue involvement and central necrosis intermediate on T1 and hyperintense on post contrast enhanced image.

Pathology
General
- Etiology-Pathogenesis
  - Aggressive neoplasms with tendency to recur and metastasize

Gross Pathologic or Surgical Features
- Unencapsulated, deep-seated tumor mass, firmly attached to adjacent deep structures
- Fleshy to hard consistency with focal areas of hemorrhage and necrosis
- Size at diagnosis usually over 5 cm

Microscopic Features
- Fibroblast like spindle cells and giant cells resembling histiocytes in pleomorphic-storiform pattern
- Necrotic foci common
- Closely resembles high-grade fibrosarcoma

Clinical Issues
Presentation
- Age: 10-90 years, peak age: 50 years, M>F
- More frequent in Caucasians
- Large, painless, soft-tissue mass with progressive enlargement over several months
- Any deep-seated, invasive, intramuscular mass in a patient >50 years is most likely MFH
- Local recurrence: 44%
- Metastases (lung, lymph nodes, liver): 42%

Treatment & Prognosis
- Surgical resection with wide margins
- Neoadjuvant and adjuvant chemotherapy in selected cases
- 5 year mortality: 55%

Malignant Fibrous Histiocytoma

Selected References
1. Murphey MD et al: From the archives of the AFIP. Musculoskeletal malignant fibrous histiocytoma: Radiologic-pathologic correlation. Radiographics. 14:807-26, 1994
2. Ros PR et al: Malignant fibrous histiocytoma: Mesenchymal tumor of ubiquitous origin. AJR. 142:753-9, 1984

Synovial Sarcoma

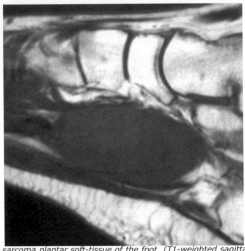

Synovial sarcoma plantar soft-tissue of the foot (T1-weighted sagittal image).

Key Facts
- Represents 8-10% of soft tissue sarcomas

Imaging Findings
General Features
- Extremities (83%), most commonly around knee and foot
- Trunk, head and neck region
- Arises from juxta-articular soft tissue, tendon sheath, rarely from joint cavity (<10%)

Plain Film Findings
- Well-defined soft-tissue mass close to joint
- Amorphous calcifications (25-30%)
- Bone invasion (10-20%): Periosteal reaction, invasion of cortex with wide zone of transition
- Juxta-articular osteoporosis

MR Findings
- T1 MR: Inhomogeneous septated mass with low SI
- T2 MR: Inhomogeneous mass with increased SI
- Infiltrative margins, fluid-fluid levels

Differential Diagnosis
Soft Tissue Chondrosarcoma
- Arises in proximal part of extremities and buttocks
- Aggressive appearance with invasion of adjacent skeletal structures

Myositis Ossificans
- Distinctive zoning phenomenon

PVNS
- Rarely calcifies

Pathology
General
- Etiology-Pathogenesis

Synovial Sarcoma

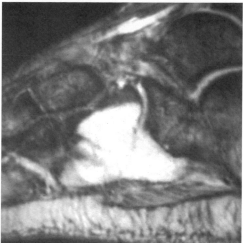

Secondary cuboid destruction with synovial sarcoma soft-tissue extension (T2* weighted sagittal image).

- ○ Tumor of high malignancy but slow growth
- ○ Does NOT arise from synovial tissue
- ○ Most tumors occur extraarticular
- ○ Originate from pluripotent mesenchyme of the limb bud

Gross Pathologic or Surgical Features
- • Solid, sharply-circumscribed mass of fleshy tissue
- • Cut surface may present areas of necrosis or hemorrhage
- • Occasional spotty areas of calcification

Microscopic Features
- • Biphasic type most common: Fibrous and epithelial component
- • Spindle and epithelial cells arranged in glandular or nest-like structure
- • Foci of calcification usually in areas of hyalinization within spindle cell element of tumor

Clinical Issues

Presentation
- • Age: 16-36, mean age: 32 years, M=F
- • Soft-tissue swelling and progressive pain
- • Soft-tissue mass, tender on palpation
- • Metastasizes to lung

Treatment & Prognosis
- • Wide surgical excision
- • High-grade lesions: Radical resection and radiation therapy
- • Chemotherapy in metastatic cases
- • High recurrence rate
- • 5 year survival: 25-55%

Selected References
1. Jones BC et al: Synovial sarcoma: MR imaging findings in 34 patients. AJR. 161:827-30, 1993
2. Morton MJ et al: MR imaging of synovial sarcoma. AJR. 156:337-40, 1991

Index of Diagnoses

NOTES

NOTES

NOTES

NOTES